Autism

Practical Knowledge and Parenting Techniques to Transform Your Explosive Child Now

(The Chaotic Symphony of a Late-diagnosed Woman's Mind)

Victor Finley

Published By **Tyson Maxwell**

Victor Finley

Autism: Practical Knowledge and Parenting Techniques to Transform Your Explosive Child Now (The Chaotic Symphony of a Late-diagnosed Woman's Mind)

ISBN   978-1-7780570-8-3

Legal & Disclaimer

Table Of Contents

Chapter 1: What Exactly Is "Autism?"

One of the largest questions about autism spectrum ailment is how it's miles added on. By searching at this line of inquiry, you can have a look at awesome theories regarding the etiology of autism and associated problems. You may additionally moreover furthermore learn about particular controversies, at the aspect of whether or not or now not or now not autism is an outgrowth of particular parenting styles, whether or not it's far associated with vaccines containing mercury, and whether or not it's far greater everyday specially racial or socioeconomic organizations. Researching this question will prepare you to talk intelligently with mother and father who've questions about their infant's evaluation.

Autism Spectrum Disorder (ASD) is a neurological and developmental illness that influences a person's capacity to talk, have interaction with others, and behave because it ought to be in social conditions. It is a spectrum sickness, which means that signs and signs and symptoms and symptoms and severity can range substantially from one person to the subsequent. Common trends of autism encompass trouble with social interaction, impaired verbal and nonverbal communique, and repetitive behaviors. People with ASD may also additionally experience problems with sensory processing, along side an aversion to loud noises or an immoderate sensitivity to touch. Additionally, humans with autism may additionally experience problem with transitions, reading new capabilities, and growing relationships. While there may be no diagnosed remedy for autism, early intervention and treatment can assist human beings with ASD learn how to control their signs and symptoms and signs and lead healthful, unbiased lives.

Autism is a complicated neurodevelopmental disorder that is believed to be due to a mixture of genetic and environmental factors. A amount of diverse genes were related to autism, and some environmental factors, which incorporates advanced parental age or publicity to excessive pleasant chemical compounds during being pregnant, may additionally moreover growth the hazard of autism. However, the right reasons of autism are despite the fact that unknown, and studies into the reasons is ongoing.

EXPERIENCING THE CULTURE (AUTISM)

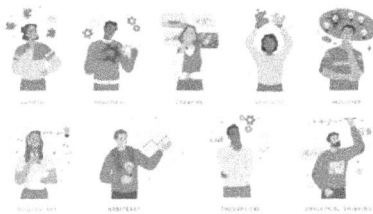

As it's miles regarded Autism is a neurological disorder that impacts someone's capability to speak and engage with others. It is a complex condition that influences all of us in each other manner, and it's far critical to understand the lifestyle surrounding autism so one can assist the ones affected. Experiencing the way of life of autism, manner gaining a better information of the studies of these dwelling with autism. It consists of gaining knowledge of approximately the stressful situations faced via way of the use of those residing with autism and the belongings available to them. It furthermore approach gaining knowledge of the unique methods in which people with autism perceive and interpret the area around them. By analyzing about the way of life of autism, you can grow to be extra privy to the language and behaviors utilized by those residing with autism, similarly to the approaches wherein they will be supported in their every day lives. Some of the ways of experiencing the life-style of autism are listed below:

Realize that autistic people make autistic tradition—no longer non-autistic humans.

Knowing that, it's far a spectrum illness; this means that that there can be a large form of symptoms and signs and symptoms, severities, and practical stages among humans with autism. Autistic people have many particular characteristics and memories, and a lifestyle has emerged from the ones shared critiques.

Autistic manner of life is notable from different cultures, and it is important to apprehend that autistic people are the simplest ones who can truely represent and apprehend autistic lifestyle. Autistic humans have a completely unique angle at the area, and this attitude has a right away impact on the cultural norms, values, and attitudes that emerge. They have their private processes of expressing themselves and navigating the arena spherical them; and non-autistic people cannot absolutely understand or recognize those reminiscences.

Non-autistic people can, but, understand and assist the autistic subculture that is created and maintained by way of manner of autistic human beings. Non-autistic human beings can use their privilege to create a more inclusive and understanding society. This manner being attentive to, believing, and respecting autistic human beings, and not making assumptions or judgments based totally definitely totally on their conduct. It also approach mastering more about autism and the memories of autistic human beings, truly so non-autistic people can higher recognize, empathize, and assist them. Ultimately, it's far crucial to understand that autistic humans are those who create and maintain autistic way of life. Non-autistic people need to attempt to create an surroundings this is accepting of autistic lifestyle and respectful of autistic humans. By doing this, we're capable of make certain that autistic lifestyle is reliable and that each one autistic humans are capable of stay first-rate, huge lives.

Go to autism-nice hashtags online.

If you are looking to connect to others who're on the autism spectrum, autism-exquisite hashtags on-line can be a beneficial device.

From on line assist businesses and fundraisers to artwork and advocacy, hashtags deliver autistic humans a platform to percent their opinions and hook up with every other.

Hashtags are a manner of labeling posts and comments on social media systems like Twitter, Instagram and Facebook. They are used to company topics and content material cloth collectively in order that clients can without difficulty discover them. By collectively with a hashtag to a post, you can right away hook up with one-of-a-kind oldsters which are talking approximately the same problem count.

For autistic human beings, autism-nice hashtags can be a terrific way to discover people who recognize and might relate to their reviews. They can locate assist, recommendation, and sources from considered one of a type parents which are at the autism spectrum, further to be part of conversations and share their memories.

Read autism-excellent books written via autistic human beings and allies. Find distinguished voices within the autistic nearby location or network

Reading books written by using way of autistic people and allies is an first rate manner to gain notion into the autistic revel in. It's a useful possibility to look at the perfect troubles that the ones at the autism spectrum face, similarly to the thrill and triumphs that come from being a part of this numerous organization. Autism-pleasant books can take many paperwork, from fiction to non-fiction, from picture books to younger individual literature. In addition to offering an statistics of autism, those books can serve as a supply of idea and instance for autistic readers. When seeking out books on autism thru autistic people and allies, it's essential to find distinguished voices in the autistic network. Autistic authors, activists, and advocates are the super property of information approximately autism, and their paintings can offer an invaluable angle at the scenario.

Fiction books via autistic authors are a awesome manner to study the lived evaluations of autistic humans. These books often draw on the writer's private research, giving readers a completely particular notion into the autistic revel in. Additionally, these books can provide a enormous deliver of instance for autistic readers. Non-fiction books thru autistic authors also are a incredible manner to take a look at autism. These books regularly provide a scholarly exploration of autism, exploring the concern thru the author's personal lens. Autistic authors also are capable of provide a completely unique perspective at the problem that may be lacking from wonderful sources. In addition to books with the aid of using using autistic authors, there are books written through allies of the autistic community. Allies can offer a beneficial mind-set on autism, exploring the venture from an out of doors aspect of view.

These books can provide perception into how neurotypical people view autism, further to how they are able to satisfactory assist autistic people. Reading autism-exceptional books written with the resource of autistic humans and allies is an important part of understanding the autistic experience. These books can provide valuable notion into the challenges and joys of being at the autism spectrum, in addition to offer a widespread deliver of instance for autistic readers. By looking for awesome voices inside the autistic community, readers can advantage a extra statistics of autism and better assist autistic people.

Reading this superb books written with the aid of way of autistic humans and their allies is one of the brilliant methods to investigate extra approximately autism and gain belief into the opinions of those residing with it. Not most effective do those books assist to raise focus and facts of autism, additionally they offer a completely unique thoughts-set that would help to bridge the space among the neurotypical and autistic organizations.

Autistic authors and allies had been sharing their recollections for years, and there may be a wealth of books to be had for those seeking out to analyze greater approximately autism. From private memoirs and biographies to fiction, the ones books offer pretty some perspectives on the autism revel in.

Many of those authors are awesome voices inside the autistic community, strolling to unfold recognition and attractiveness of autism. These books may be a outstanding beneficial aid for those attempting to find to benefit a deeper facts of autism and its effect on those residing with it, further to their households and loved ones. They can also offer valuable perception into the struggles and successes of autistic people, and how they navigate their lives and the area round them. By analyzing those books, readers can advantage a better appreciation of the correct demanding situations and presents related to autism, and advantage a better knowledge of the manner to help and engage with autistic human beings.

There are some of prominent autistic authors and allies who have written books approximately their tales. Among the maximum well-known are Naoki Higashida, writer of The Reason I Jump, and John Elder Robison, author of Look Me inside the Eye. Other incredible authors encompass Ido Kedar, writer of The Autistic Brain, and Temple Grandin, author of Thinking in Pictures. In addition to books written with the resource of the usage of autistic authors, there also are some of books written thru allies who've near connections to the autistic community.

These books offer a useful aid for the ones searching out to higher understand autism and the evaluations of these dwelling with it. Some of these authors embody Alix Generous, creator of Neurodivergent, and Steve Silberman, writer of NeuroTribes. Reading books written through autistic people and their allies is an crucial manner to boom recognition and information of autism. By learning extra about the unique studies of these residing with autism, readers can gain a more appreciation for the complexity of the disability and the energy of those suffering from it. Additionally, the ones books can help to bridge the gap the various neurotypical and autistic groups and manual the beauty of autism in all its forms.

Mark autism sports for your calendar and Participate in autism-related occasions.

Autism spectrum illness (ASD) is a complicated neurodevelopmental sickness that impacts humans in masses of strategies. As a surrender quit end result, developing recognition and information of ASD is surprisingly essential. One of the great techniques to do this is to mark autism sports to your calendar and take part in autism-related occasions. Marking autism sports on your calendar is a exceptional way to live updated with the current statistics and data about ASD. There are many sports during the twelve months which might be committed to instructing humans approximately autism and supplying beneficial aid for those involved. These occasions can be held in character or surely, and may include meetings, movie screenings, art work exhibitions, and extra.

Participating in autism-associated sports is an terrific manner to show your assist and determination to elevating interest and information of autism. It additionally offers you an opportunity to study more about the sickness and connect to humans of the autism community. You can discover autism events to mark in your calendar for your community community, on-line, or thru businesses that provide help for those stricken by autism. Participating in the ones occasions also can assist you assemble relationships with other humans within the autism community.

Marking autism activities in your calendar and taking detail in autism-associated activities is an vital way to assist spread popularity, elegance and understanding of autism. Doing so will help create a more inclusive and understanding environment for human beings affected by ASD, and may make a difference in their lives.

Learn the commonplace terminology to keep away from terrible language at the identical time as speaking with autistic people

When talking with an autistic man or woman, it's miles critical to bear in mind of the language used and to avoid the usage of horrible language. People with autism regularly have problem interpreting and responding to language inside the same way as people who aren't on the spectrum, so the use of language that is not in all likelihood to be misinterpreted is vital for growing a great and green communique. To make sure that conversations are terrific and beneficial for all worried, it's miles essential to be familiar with the not unusual terminology used whilst discussing autism. The time period "autism spectrum sickness" (ASD) is used to explain a lot of conditions that have an effect on communique and social interaction.

AUTISM IS A NEUROLOGICAL DISORDER THAT IS OFTEN CHARACTERIZED BY DIFFICULTY INTERPRETING SOCIAL CUES, REPETITIVE BEHAVIORS, AND DIFFICULTY WITH COMMUNICATION.

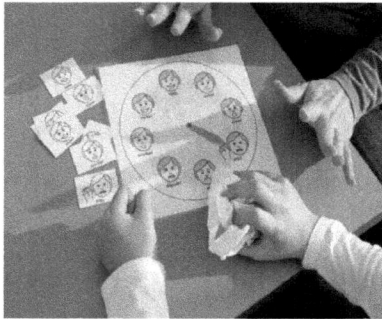

It is vital to avoid using language which means that autism is a incapacity or that humans with autism are "DISABLED". Instead, it's far greater suitable to use language that means that autism is a difference and that people with autism have specific skills and strengths.

The term "NEURODIVERSITY" is regularly used to describe the idea that neurological versions want to be celebrated and regular. It is vital to avoid the usage of language that implies that people with autism are "ABNORMAL" or

"DEFICIENT". Instead, it is higher to use language that means that people with autism are "DIFFERENT" and that their neurological variations should be embraced.

The term "ACCOMMODATIONS" is used to give an explanation for the strategies, techniques, and permits which is probably used to assist individuals with autism to better participate in sports, capabilities, and sports activities. It is crucial to keep away from using language which means that that individuals with autism want to be "FIXED" OR "CURED". Instead, it is greater appropriate to apply language that means that individuals with autism require guide and lodges as a way to obtain their capability.

The term "INCLUSION" is used to give an explanation for a motion that encourages people with autism to be included in all components of existence. It is vital to avoid using language meaning that human beings with autism need to be "EXCLUDED" OR "ISOLATED". Instead, it's miles greater appropriate to use language that means that human beings with autism need to have the equal opportunities and be protected in all factors of life.

The term "NEURODIVERSITY POSITIVE" is used to offer an explanation for strategies and attitudes that emphasize the strengths and abilties of humans with autism. It is vital to keep away from the use of language that means that humans with autism are "INFERIOR" OR "UNWANTED". Instead, it is extra appropriate to use language that means that human beings with autism should be well-known and revered for their specific abilities and strengths.

By familiarizing yourself with those phrases and retaining off horrible language whilst speakme with an autistic man or woman, you could help to create a incredible and effective communique. Being conscious of the language used can help to make certain that conversations ARE RESPECTFUL,

MEANINGFUL, AND BENEFICIAL for all concerned or concerned.

Learn approximately excessive fantastic and horrible symbols associated with autism and take note of how autistic people describe autism.

As a stop end end result, the symbols and imagery associated with autism can be each high quality and negative. Positive symbols related to autism ought to likely include PUZZLES, as they constitute the complexity of the ailment and the man or woman's journey to knowledge it. Another fantastic photo is a RAINBOW; that is regularly used to represent variety and inclusion.

Artwork and photos of kids with autism additionally may be visible as a effective photograph, highlighting the power and creativity of autistic people. Negative symbols related to autism may additionally additionally encompass a PUZZLE PIECE, this is regularly visible as a image of the sickness's complexity and the dearth of statistics that also surrounds it. Another terrible photo is a person's arms protecting their ears, that is regularly used to symbolize the demanding situations that autistic individuals face close to sensory overload.

It's moreover crucial to be aware of how autistic humans describe autism. Every autistic individual opinions autism in some different manner, so it's important to understand their views on the disease. Some also can furthermore view autism as a "SUPERPOWER" OR A "GIFT", on the identical time as others can also view it as a "CHALLENGE OR A DISABILITY". Every character is unique, so it's crucial to be open to all views.

Ultimately, it's essential to recognize that the symbols related to autism are both incredible and bad. It's essential to have in thoughts of the messages that the ones symbols send, and to be respectful of the perspectives of autistic individuals. By information the tremendous and horrific symbols associated with autism, we can art work to create a more inclusive and understanding international for the ones on the autism spectrum.

Consult autistic human beings and discover approximately common misconceptions about autism.

Autism is a complicated and regularly misunderstood state of affairs that impacts the lives of many people from all walks of lifestyles. While there's but a first rate deal to be located out approximately autism, there are some commonplace misconceptions that may be addressed with the useful resource of speaking with autistic human beings and studying greater approximately their opinions.

Chapter 2: Autism "Awareness" & Autism "Acceptance"

Autism interest is a developing problem throughout the world. It is predicted that 1 in 59 children are diagnosed with autism spectrum contamination (ASD). Autism is a complex neurological sickness that impacts how a person communicates and interacts with others. Those with autism often experience hassle in social interplay, repetitive behaviors, and sensory issues. It is essential to raise cognizance about autism so that you can higher understand the sickness and assist those affected.

Education is one of the key to know-how autism and getting to know the way to higher useful useful resource humans with the sickness. It is likewise critical to create an inclusive environment for those with autism and provide possibilities for them to take part in sports activities sports that are large to them. One manner to create autism popularity is to train others approximately the ailment. This can embody imparting information approximately the signs and symptoms and signs and symptoms and signs and symptoms and signs of autism, sharing tales of people with autism, and supplying belongings and help.

It is likewise essential to understand the variety of autism and its results on every individual. Creating an inclusive surroundings is a few other way to promote autism recognition. This can encompass presenting sensory-fine areas, making motels for people with autism, and creating social and leisure sports activities which is probably welcoming and to be had to people with ASD.

Autism reputation also involves advocating for those with autism. This can embody advocating for higher services and assets, advocating for greater inclusive training and healthcare, and advocating for the rights of people with autism (This is probably high-quality stated later in distinctive chapters).

Finally, it's miles vital to bear in mind that people with autism are just like all of us else.

They need to be handled with respect and kindness and given the same possibilities that everyone else has. Raising autism recognition can assist create an surroundings in which people with autism sense common and supported. It can also assist to reduce the stigma and discrimination related to autism. With prolonged statistics, beauty, and guide, humans with autism can gather their whole ability.

Autism "reputation" is a time period that is used to seek advice from the idea of making an inclusive society for humans with autism. It is prepared knowledge, valuing, and embracing the particular developments of humans with autism, further to the ability they ought to make contributions to the arena. Autism recognition calls for us to appearance past the traditional view of autism as a disability that wishes to be "FIXED" OR "CURED," and rather awareness at the "ABILITIES AND STRENGTHS" of people with autism.

It is ready recognizing that humans with autism are part of our network and are entitled to the equal rights and recognize as a few exclusive man or woman. It way recognizing that autism is a clearly happening difference, and it's far our obligation to create a society this is inclusive, supportive, and empowering for people with autism.

The idea of autism recognition is going in addition than in fact recognizing the lifestyles of autism or autism attention. It consists of actively going for walks to create a worldwide this is welcoming and supportive of human beings with autism. This manner that we should try to create companies and environments which is probably to be had and accommodating to humans with autism, so that it will participate genuinely in society.

It consists of imparting massive opportunities for humans with autism to specific themselves and to pursue their passions and interests. It moreover consists of information the unique needs and annoying conditions of people with autism, and operating to create powerful and appropriate supports and offerings to fulfill their desires.

The idea of autism beauty is gaining traction in lots of groups round the world. It is a motion that is bringing together humans from all walks of lifestyles to create a greater inclusive and knowledge society for humans with autism. By embracing this concept, we're capable of make certain that everyone with autism has the hazard to stay a full and widespread life.

DIFFERENCE BETWEEN AUTISM AWARENESS AND AUTISM ACCEPTANCE

The difference amongst autism cognizance and autism recognition is that attention is the understanding and understanding of autism, whilst elegance is the confirmation and appreciation of people with autism and the price they carry approximately about to society.

AUTISM AWARENESS is the first step in expertise the ailment. It's critical to recognize the signs and symptoms and symptoms and signs of autism, in addition to the property available to people with autism and their families. Awareness moreover helps to lessen the stigma associated with autism and create a greater accepting environment for human beings with autism.

AUTISM ACCEPTANCE, as a substitute, is set going beyond consciousness. It includes recognizing and appreciating the specific abilities of humans with autism, and accepting them for who they'll be. Acceptance additionally way spotting that everybody has the right to be dealt with with dignity and understand, irrespective of their skills or disabilities. When discussing autism popularity, it's far vital to understand that there are a whole lot of strategies that humans with autism can be customary into society. This includes supplying suitable educational and employment possibilities, further to providing get proper of access to to social sports and leisure possibilities.

It is likewise vital to understand that humans with autism may want to have significant relationships and friendships, and to create an surroundings in which they may experience ordinary and valued.

Autism attention is an critical a part of information and reducing the stigma related to autism, however reputation is the essential factor to growing an inclusive and supportive surroundings for humans with autism. Acceptance manner recognizing the cost and ability of sincerely all and sundry, no matter their abilties or disabilities. It moreover manner knowledge that everybody has the proper to be everyday and respected, and being willing to make resorts to make sure that people with autism can take part in all elements of lifestyles.

NOTE: The difference among autism AWARENESS and ACCEPTANCE is that attention is the know-how and know-how of the ailment, WHILE splendor is the popularity and appreciation of people with autism and the rate they bring about about to society.

Awareness is an important first step, but it's miles Acceptance that creates a more inclusive and supportive environment. Only via recognition can human beings with autism be simply included in society and be able to reap their entire capability.

RELATING WITH AUTISTIC PEOPLE

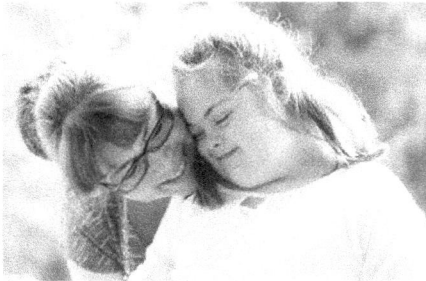

Autism is a complicated and varied state of affairs, and every body with autism is one-of-a-kind. As such, there can be no man or woman-duration-suits-all method to interacting with autistic human beings.

However, there are sure suggestions that might assist make the interplay extra a hit.

Autism! As it's far called a neurological sickness that would have a incredible effect on how someone pertains to others. It impacts the manner someone communicates, acts, and interacts with distinct people. Autistic people regularly have hassle knowledge the social cues of others, that might make it difficult for them to hook up with the ones round them. With the right help, but, autistic people can study to relate to others in huge strategies. One of the most important matters even as relating to autistic humans is to be affected person and data. Autistic humans can also take longer to manner information, or might not be able to speak their thoughts in the equal manner as someone without autism. It is crucial to be affected man or woman and supply them the time they want to answer to a state of affairs. It is likewise vital to be aware of the individual's strengths and weaknesses.

Autistic humans have a sizeable sort of abilties and demanding situations, and it's miles critical to be aware of the ones at the identical time as relating to them. This will assist you understand their conduct and reply because of this. Another vital aspect to preserve in thoughts is to be aware about sensory sensitivities. Autistic people can be touchy to first rate sounds, smells, and textures, and it is crucial to be aware about this on the identical time as speaking with them. It is likewise important to be aware of their need for habitual and shape, and to be bendy whilst essential. When communicating with autistic human beings, it's far critical to use language this is easy and direct.

Autistic human beings may additionally moreover moreover have issue expertise subtlety or sarcasm, so it's miles vital to be particular and avoid using metaphors or figures of speech. When it comes to physical contact, it's miles essential to be aware of the individual's comfort level. Autistic people may not enjoy physical contact or can also find it overwhelming, so it is vital to be privy to this while concerning them. It is also critical to be aware of the character's pastimes and wishes. Autistic humans may also have very specific hobbies and dreams, and it is critical to be privy to the ones even as interacting with them. This allow you to find out common pastimes and activities that you could every revel in.

Finally, it's miles important to reveal recognize and attractiveness. Autistic humans have the same smooth want and goals as everyone else, and they want to be dealt with with recognize and recognition. Showing recognize and recognition can assist create a tremendous dating among you and an autistic character. Relating to autistic people can be difficult, however it can furthermore be profitable. With staying electricity, data, and appreciate, it's miles possible to build massive relationships with autistic people. By records their dreams and annoying conditions, and displaying apprehend and recognition, you can create a high-quality dating that is beneficial for both of you. Try those techniques of concerning with them:

1. BE PATIENT: Patience is a key element whilst interacting with autistic humans. It can take humans with autism longer to method and respond to questions and remarks. They can also want greater time to anticipate and respond.

Autism is a complex developmental illness that influences someone's capability to interact and speak with others. It is a spectrum disorder, because of this that the severity of the disease can range from man or woman to character. People with autism can experience problem in social conditions and verbal exchange, in addition to have limited hobbies and repetitive conduct. The specific cause of autism is unknown, but it is believed to be a mixture of genetic and environmental factors.

There isn't any therapy for autism, however early intervention and remedy can help enhance the signs and help the character lead a extra independent existence. It is essential to recognize that no   human beings with autism are alike. They may have comparable signs and symptoms, however the manner they explicit them and the severity of the symptoms can range.

They may also have trouble with social skills, conversation, and expertise unique people's perspectives. They can also have hassle with sensory processing, similarly to problems with motor skills. When demanding for a person with autism, it's miles crucial to be expertise and affected man or woman. It is important not to determine their conduct and to apprehend their feelings. It is likewise critical to be privy to their triggers and to avoid them if possible.

It is critical to do not forget that people with autism can however shape big relationships and lead efficient lives. With the right beneficial aid and interventions, people with autism can examine the manner to speak and have interaction with others in massive strategies. When interacting with a person with autism, it's miles essential to be affected character and know-how. It is crucial to provide them time to way statistics and to recognize what they may be attempting to say. It is likewise critical to apply clean and easy language and to keep away from jargon or slang. It is also important to be aware about their sensory sensitivities. Some human beings with autism may be touchy to noise, contact, or high quality smells. It is critical to be aware about those sensitivities and to make lodges if critical.

It is also vital to offer shape and consistency. People with autism may additionally need help understanding the expectations that are positioned on them and might need help following via with duties. It is essential to provide guide and encouragement at the same time as they learn how to control their conduct.

Finally, it is crucial to provide sizeable sports activities and possibilities for learning. People with autism may also moreover moreover need help information the arena spherical them and locating ways to have interaction in excellent sports activities. It is essential to provide sports activities which may be every fun and academic. Caring for someone with autism can be tough, but it can moreover be very worthwhile. With staying energy and information, it's miles possible to offer the assist and help that human beings with autism need to guide a fulfillment and enjoyable lives.

2. PROVIDE STRUCTURE: Autistic human beings often understand structure and normal. Providing an surroundings with easy expectancies and policies can help purpose them to enjoy more cushty.

Providing shape for an autistic character may be a hard project, as autism is a neurological contamination that impacts how someone interacts with their environment. Autistic human beings regularly warfare with information and following the expectations of others, making it hard to create a established surroundings. However, with some smooth strategies and an statistics of the manner autism impacts someone's behavior and development, imparting shape for an autistic person can be completed.

The first step in presenting form for an autistic individual is to understand their man or woman desires. Autism impacts everyone in a few other way, so it's critical to get to recognise the person and their precise strengths and weaknesses. This will help you create a form this is tailored to their specific goals. Additionally, it's crucial to understand that supplying form for an autistic man or woman can be an extended-time period technique, because the character may additionally moreover require specific tiers of assist as they develop and increase. Once you have got a better facts of the individual's dreams, you can begin to create a form.

A precise vicinity to begin is to create a each day normal. Autistic human beings regularly thrive on recurring, because it gives them a sense of safety and predictability. Set a ordinary time table for meals, sports activities, and bedtime, and attempt to persist with it as lots as possible. Additionally, wreck down duties into small, doable steps and use visible cues, like a timeline or chart, to assist the character recognize what is anticipated of them.

When presenting form for an autistic character, it's important to preserve the surroundings as calm and prepared as possible. Minimize distractions and loud noises, and provide a quiet, cushty location for the person to retreat to in the occasion that they end up crushed. Additionally, make certain to give the man or woman hundreds of splendid reinforcement, and provide visible cues and reminders to assist them recognize what is predicted of them.

Finally, it's essential to consider that presenting shape for an autistic person is an ongoing device. As the individual grows and develops, their dreams can also moreover change, and you can want to regulate the shape therefore. Additionally, ensure to be affected character and understanding; autism can be a hard sickness to govern, and it's essential to expose compassion and recognition. With the right help and shape, an autistic character can thrive

three. BE RESPECTFUL: Respect is critical at the equal time as interacting with autistic people. Speak to them as you'll absolutely everyone else and keep away from making assumptions approximately their abilties or hobbies.

Being respectful to an autistic character is an vital a part of making them revel in snug and time-honored in society. Autistic people are often misunderstood and mistreated because of their variations in verbal exchange and conduct. As a forestall quit result, it's far essential to be privy to the annoying conditions that autistic people also can furthermore face and to be respectful and facts of them. Autism is a neurodevelopmental state of affairs that affects how someone interacts with the vicinity and the manner they gadget facts. People at the autism spectrum can also additionally have hassle with conversation, social interaction, and conduct. They may have sensory sensitivities, that might make it hard to respond to high quality people or situations in a normal manner. As a end result, it is vital to be respectful while interacting with an autistic character.

This manner being affected character and information after they battle to talk, fending off making assumptions about their conduct, and not making any judgments. It is likewise important to be aware of their sensory sensitivities and to recognize of the environment that they're in. Making sure to include an autistic individual in conversations and sports activities is likewise crucial. Autistic people can also have problem information or assignment conversations, so it's far important to provide them with the opportunity to take part.

It is also important to be aware about any triggers that would reason them to grow to be crushed or dissatisfied, and to be understanding and supportive if this occurs. It is likewise vital to be privy to how an autistic person can be feeling. Autistic people may not be able to specific their emotions inside the identical manner as neurotypical human beings, so it's far critical to be privy to any changes in their behavior or temper. If an autistic individual appears to be struggling, it's far crucial to be respectful and supportive in preference to judgmental or important.

Finally, it is important to recognize an autistic man or woman's obstacles. Autistic human beings may additionally additionally want greater time and area to method their emotions and opinions. As a quit result, it is crucial to consider of their desires and to appreciate any boundaries that they've set. Respecting an autistic character is important for making them enjoy standard and supported. Autistic humans regularly face stressful situations in communique and behavior, and it is important to be aware of those traumatic situations and to be respectful and facts of them. By being respectful and supportive, we are capable of help create an environment in which autistic people experience stable and common.

four. BE OPEN TO DIFFERENT WAYS OF COMMUNICATION:

Autistic human beings might also moreover furthermore talk in brilliant strategies. They can also moreover use non-verbal cues together with facial expressions or frame language, or they may use opportunity types of verbal exchange which includes picture change or signal language.

Communication is a important part of human interaction and it's far vital to constructing relationships. However, information the way to efficiently talk with someone who has autism isn't constantly easy. Autistic human beings expect and manner information in any other case than neurotypical people, so even as speaking with them, it's miles crucial to be aware of their specific needs. Autism is a neurological disorder that affects how someone communicates and interacts with others. It is characterised through deficits in social interplay, conversation, and behavior.

People with autism ought to have trouble data and expressing their emotions, in addition to issue records and interpreting the feelings of others. When speaking with an autistic person, it's far important to be open to particular methods of communication. Autistic humans can also have issue talking within the identical techniques that neurotypical humans do.

People with autism regularly have trouble knowledge frame language and facial expressions, so it is crucial to talk in methods which is probably greater direct and open. One manner to efficiently talk with an autistic person is to offer verbal cues; This can encompass offering clean instructions, setting expectancies, and the usage of easy language. It is likewise critical to be affected man or woman and provide the person time to approach the information.

Another way to speak with an autistic man or woman is to use seen cues. Visual aids along side photographs, diagrams, and films may be very beneficial for autistic individuals who've trouble expertise verbal communication. Visual cues can help autistic humans better apprehend the data that is being communicated. When talking with an autistic character, it's far important to be privy to their sensory sensitivities. Autistic human beings can be sensitive to sure sounds, smells, and textures. It is important to be aware about any sensitivities and to avoid overwhelming the individual with too much information right now.

It is likewise crucial to be aware about the person's stage of understanding. Autistic humans can also moreover additionally have problem expertise and interpreting language, so it's miles critical to be affected character and use clean language at the same time as speaking.

Finally, it's miles important to be aware about the manner you talk with an autistic man or woman. Autistic humans can be very sensitive to criticism and awful feedback, so it is vital to talk in a supportive and inspiring manner. Communicating with an autistic man or woman may be a undertaking, however it's far essential to be open to awesome techniques of conversation. By being aware of the character's precise desires, speaking in a supportive manner, and the usage of seen and verbal cues, it's miles possible to create an effective and massive conversation.

five. USE SIMPLE LANGUAGE: Autistic human beings may additionally additionally additionally find it difficult to understand complex language. Try to apply clean language and keep away from prolonged, complicated sentences.

Autism is a complicated neurological disorder this is characterized through trouble in communication, social interaction, and sensory integration. Autism is a lifelong situation that influences a person's capability to engage and communicate with others. It can range from slight to immoderate and might affect a person in a single-of-a-type strategies. People with autism can also have problem knowledge and expressing themselves. They may have trouble information others, social cues, and forming relationships. They can also revel in sensory overload, because of this they may be resultseasily crushed with the aid of using way of loud noises, vibrant lighting fixtures, and special sensory stimuli.

People with autism may additionally furthermore need greater time and workout to analyze new abilities. They can be slower to research language, have trouble with motor talents, and conflict to narrate to others. People with autism also can have hassle knowledge extraordinary human beings's emotions and emotions.

It is normally diagnosed in kids most of the some time of two and six. However, it is able to be recognized at any age. It is vital to word that autism is not a one-length-fits-all state of affairs and anybody's revel in with autism is specific.

There is not any recognised treatment for autism, but there are various remedies and interventions which could assist enhance the lives of humans with autism. These remedies and interventions can assist people with autism find out procedures to speak, deal with sensory overload, and construct relationships. Behavioral treatment is one of the maximum commonplace treatments for autism. This form of therapy makes a speciality of training human beings with autism a manner to interact and speak in social conditions.

It also can help them learn how to manipulate their feelings, similarly to enhance their language, motor, and hassle-solving competencies. Other treatments and interventions for autism consist of speech-language treatment, occupational remedy, and treatment. Speech-language remedy can help humans with autism beautify their verbal exchange capabilities.

OCCUPATIONAL THERAPY can assist people with autism enhance their motor competencies and sensory integration. Additionally, medicinal tablets may be used to help manage difficult behaviors associated with autism. Autism is a lifelong circumstance, however human beings with autism can live glad and exciting lives. With the right supports and interventions, humans with autism can discover ways to speak, socialize, and extend full-size relationships. It is vital to bear in mind that autism is not a one-length-suits-all condition and every body's enjoy with autism is precise.

6. Avoid Overstimulation: Autistic people can be effortlessly overstimulated, so it's miles

crucial to keep away from overwhelming them with too much records immediately.

Overstimulation is one of the maximum not unusual problems skilled through using human beings with autism. It can occur itself in physical, behavioral, and emotional approaches. It also can have an effect on social and communication abilities. Overstimulation is regularly due to sensory overload, which occurs while the senses have trouble processing and responding to all the incoming stimuli. When human beings with autism become overstimulated, they'll display signs and symptoms and signs and symptoms of physical tension, collectively with clenching their fists or rocking from side to side. They can also show signs and symptoms and signs of emotional misery, inclusive of becoming agitated or overreacting to a situation.

Overstimulation can also result in modifications in conduct, consisting of keeping off social situations or becoming overly competitive. In order to keep away from overstimulation with autistic human beings, it's miles important to create a secure and comfortable environment. This manner avoiding loud noises, shiny lights, and distinctive sensory triggers that can motive overstimulation. It is also essential to be aware of the person's person wishes and possibilities, as those also can range from individual to character. It is essential to be aware about the signs and symptoms and signs and symptoms and symptoms of overstimulation, so you can take steps to reduce it.

These signs and symptoms and signs and symptoms can include bodily anxiety, emotional distress, adjustments in conduct, and avoidance of social situations. If you've got a look at any of those symptoms and signs and signs, it is critical to accomplish that to reduce the overstimulation. One way to reduce overstimulation is to provide a stable and snug surroundings. This can include dimming lighting, decreasing noise stages, and retaining off sensory triggers. It is also important to provide a distraction from the overstimulation. This may be a few element as clean as a coloring e-book, a puzzle, or a chilled hobby.

Another way to reduce overstimulation is to provide breaks from the environment. This can embody taking a walk outside, going to a quiet room, or undertaking calming sports activities. It is important to be privy to the individual's person desires, so that you can offer sports sports which might be calming and thrilling. It is likewise essential to provide form and everyday. Having a normal time table can assist lessen pressure and overstimulation. This can encompass having meals and sports activities activities at the identical time each day, further to providing smooth expectancies and hints. This can assist the person to feel extra secure and on pinnacle of things in their surroundings.

Finally, it's miles vital to be information and patient. People with autism may also moreover emerge as overstimulated with out problems, and it is important to be expertise of this. It is likewise important to don't forget that overstimulation may be a symptom of some issue else, and it's far crucial to are looking for for expert assist if the overstimulation is inflicting distress or impacting at the character's lifestyles.

Overstimulation may be a hard problem to control, however it is viable to reduce it and create a secure and snug surroundings for human beings with autism. By being aware about the signs and symptoms of overstimulation, presenting a steady and cushty environment, offering breaks from the surroundings, supplying form and routine, and being data and affected man or woman, it's miles viable to avoid overstimulation with autistic people.

7. Acknowledge Feelings: Autistic humans may also moreover have trouble expressing their emotions, so listen to them and let them apprehend that it's miles properly enough to have feelings.

Acknowledging an autistic individual's feelings may be an extremely profitable experience. It can assist assemble take delivery of as actual with and mutual expertise between an autistic individual and those spherical them. It also can assist construct arrogance and self belief in the autistic man or woman, as they sense seen, heard, and understood. Acknowledging an autistic person's emotions can come in many office work, including verbal and non-verbal communique. It also can encompass physical gestures which encompass a hug, pat at the again, or keeping fingers.

The first step in acknowledging an autistic character's emotions is to recognize how they are feeling and why. Autistic humans can often revel in severe emotions, and it may be tough for them to explicit their emotions. It is critical to be patient and facts at the same time as searching for to emerge as privy to what the character is feeling.

This can be done with the aid of the use of looking their frame language, facial expressions, and vocal tone. Being an active listener and asking questions on what the character is feeling also can be beneficial. Once you have identified how the individual is feeling, it's far vital to validate their emotions. This approach communicating to them that their emotions are legitimate and worth of being recounted.

Chapter 3: Advocate For Autistic People

Advocating for autistic human beings is an crucial a part of developing an inclusive society. By education your self and others, talking up even as essential, supporting autistic-led corporations, the usage of your voice, working for inclusive change, and celebrating autistic human beings, you may be an effective suggest for autistic rights.

There are numerous strategies to endorse for autistic humans 1. Educate yourself, your own family, and your friends on autism. Research what autism is, take a look at the worrying conditions and strengths of autistic people, and be open to discussing the subject with others.

2. Reach out to your representatives. Write letters, make mobile telephone calls, or agenda meetings with them to speak about the problems that autistic people face and the way our criminal pointers can better protect them.

3. Support and donate to autism charities and advocacy agencies. These agencies are committed to elevating recognition, supplying belongings, and advocating for the rights of autistic people.

4. Participate in occasions and campaigns that help autistic humans. Show your guide via the usage of attending or organizing activities, participating in rallies and marches, and spreading the message on social media.

5. Listen to and make bigger the voices of autistic humans. Follow autistic human beings on social media, study their blogs and articles, and percentage their tales to help spread consciousness.

6. Advocate for better services and property for autistic human beings. Research the offerings available to autistic human beings to your community and work to growth get right of entry to to the ones assets.

Advocating for autistic people includes advocating for their rights, reputation,

reputation and inclusion in all factors of life. This can consist of advocating for higher get right of entry to to healthcare, training, employment, and community offerings. It also includes working to lessen stigma and promoting public information of autism. Advocates can art work to make certain that autistic humans have get entry to to suitable and evidence-based absolutely interventions, which encompass "Applied Behavior Analysis (ABA) remedy".

They can also paintings to make certain that autistic humans are represented in coverage and choice-making techniques. Advocates can manual autistic humans in acquiring low fee inns in the place of business and academic settings, and in advocating for their very very personal rights. They can also artwork to ensure that autistic humans have get proper of get right of entry to to to significant and suitable facilitates and offerings in the network.

1. Understand the Challenges Autism is a complicated neurological disorder that impacts communique, social interplay, and conduct. Autistic people can also experience problem with verbal and non-verbal conversation, difficulty in social conditions, problem with sensory overload, and problem with government functioning. It is essential to recognize the disturbing situations that autistic human beings might also moreover face so one can be an effective propose.

2. Educate Yourself and Others Advocating for autistic humans can be a complicated and hard manner. It is important to stay informed approximately present day-day studies and to hold coaching yourself and others about autism. This information will allow you to increase effective strategies for advocating for people with autism.

3. Speak Up It is crucial to speak up on the equal time as you notice an autistic individual being treated unfairly or not being furnished with the property they need. This might also

additionally advise speakme to teachers, employers, or healthcare carriers to ensure that they'll be presenting appropriate care and offerings to the autistic man or woman.

4. Support Autistic-Led Organizations Autistic-led businesses are companies which can be run through autistic people and their allies. These businesses are essential assets for advocating for autistic human beings and their wishes. Support those businesses with the useful resource of using turning into a member of their mailing lists, attending their activities, and donating to their reasons.

5. Use Your Voice Advocacy for autistic humans can take many forms. You can use your voice for your network via writing letters for your network representatives and hosting activities to raise awareness approximately autism. You also can use your voice online with the aid of the use of social media to unfold popularity about autism and advocate for autistic people.

6. Work for Inclusive Change Advocacy for autistic human beings want to recognition on growing an inclusive society that recognizes the rights and desires of autistic people. This may also moreover incorporate jogging collectively with your nearby authorities to make certain that schools and public areas are reachable and inviting to autistic people.

It might also comprise advocating for recommendations that protect the rights of autistic human beings.

7. Celebrate Autistic People In addition to advocating for the rights of autistic humans, it is also critical to have an amazing time their achievements and successes. This may also encompass net web hosting events that don't forget autistic artists, musicians, and writers. It also can encompass recognizing and amplifying the voices of autistic people in well-known manner of existence.

AUTISTIC BEHAVIOUR

It is characterized with the aid of stressful conditions associated with sensory processing, repetitive behaviors, social interactions, verbal exchange, and one in all a kind regions. People with autism often exhibit behaviors that can be tough for those spherical them to recognize. Common behaviors related to autism include a loss of social interaction, hassle making eye touch, reduced interest in sports, and repetitive actions.

Autistic human beings might also moreover have trouble expressing their emotions, have issue statistics social cues, or may be not able to look at spoken commands. One of the maximum not unusual behaviors visible in human beings with autism is the want for recurring, or a inflexible shape of their every

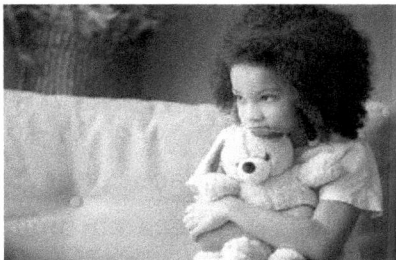

day lives.

Autistic human beings may moreover emerge as distressed or annoyed at the same time as their recurring or form is modified or disrupted. They can also become traumatic or beaten while new sports activities sports are introduced, or when they'll be predicted to perform a little thing sudden.

Other behaviors seen in people with autism encompass: - Difficulty with change: Autistic people also can have problem with transitions and might emerge as beaten or disturbing even as their normal is altered. - Repetitive behaviors: Autistic human beings may additionally have interaction in repetitive behaviors along side rocking, spinning, hand-flapping, or repeating the equal phrases or terms.

Stimming: Stimming, or self-stimulatory conduct, is a commonplace conduct visible in humans with autism. It can encompass hand-flapping, rocking, spinning, or repeating terms or phrases.

Sensory sensitivities: Autistic humans can be hypersensitive to sound, mild, or tactile sensations, or they'll be hyposensitive and now not reply to their surroundings.

Restricted interests: Autistic people may additionally have restricted interests and might turn out to be passionate about a specific challenge count or interest.

Social interplay issues: Autistic people may have problem with social interactions, which encompass starting up conversations, know-how frame language, or information social cues.

Anxiety: Autistic people may also moreover experience tension or fear because of unusual environments or situations. Autism is a spectrum disease, which means that that that the severity of signs and symptoms and signs can variety notably from individual to individual. It is essential to undergo in thoughts that autistic human beings are people, and that everyone with autism has precise dreams, behaviors, and competencies. Some conduct exhibit by means of way of autistic person can be extra defined beneath:

NOT RESPONDING TO THEIR NAME.

Autism is a situation that affects someone's functionality to technique sensory information and engage with the area around them. As a stop cease result, humans with autism might not reply to their call at the same time as referred to as. This can be a deliver of frustration and confusion for own family individuals, friends, and instructors. When someone with autism does no longer respond to their name, it is essential to undergo in mind the context and the man or woman.

There can be a number of motives why they do no longer reply, collectively with:

1. They might not have heard their name because of sensory overload. People with

autism regularly have trouble processing auditory information and won't be capable of approach their call in a loud environment.

2. They might not apprehend the idea of their call. People with autism may not recognize the which means that in their name or that it is used to are seeking recommendation from them especially.

three. They can be overwhelmed. People with autism can become crushed without problem and may not respond to their name even as they will be in an demanding or overstimulated united states.

4. They might not be geared up to have interaction. People with autism can also need more time to system social interactions and won't be ready to reply even as their call is known as.

It is crucial to take into account that it is not a lack of respect while a person with autism does not respond to their name. It is frequently due to the problems associated with autism and it's far crucial to be affected man or woman and understanding.

There are a few strategies that may be hired to help a person with autism reply to their call:

1. Use seen cues. People with autism often respond higher to visible cues than verbal ones. It can be helpful to thing to your self whilst calling their call and making sure they're searching at you.

2. Give them time to reply. It may be useful to give the character with autism time to manner their call and reply.

three. Use fantastic reinforcement. It can be beneficial to reward the person with autism when they do reply to their call. This can help improve the conduct and make it more likely they'll reply within the future. Responding to as a minimum one's call is an essential social expertise, however it is able to be difficult for people with autism. With knowledge and staying power, it's miles feasible to help a person with autism learn how to respond to their name.

AVOIDING EYE CONTACT.

Autism spectrum sickness (ASD) is a neurodevelopmental disease characterised with the useful resource of impaired social interaction, communication, and repetitive behaviors. One of the number one demanding situations for humans at the autism spectrum is hassle with interpersonal verbal exchange, which could embody averting eye contact.

Eye touch is an vital form of nonverbal verbal exchange that might sign attentiveness and interest in every different individual. For people at the autism spectrum, but, eye touch can be uncomfortable or even overwhelming. People at the autism spectrum may avoid eye touch for numerous reasons, at the side of difficulty decoding the that means of facial expressions, sensory overload, and feeling crushed via the depth of someone's gaze.

In order to higher apprehend why people with ASD may also avoid eye touch, it's far vital to examine the underlying worrying situations of autism. People with autism might also additionally additionally have problem knowledge social cues and interpreting facial expressions, that may make eye contact hard. They can also be overwhelmed via the intensity of someone's gaze and can be not capable of tolerate the sensation of being stared at.

Additionally, humans with autism can be touchy to sensory stimuli, and the near proximity of some unique person's face can be an excessive amount of for them to address. It is important to do not forget that avoiding eye touch isn't a sign of disrespect or disinterest. For individuals on the autism spectrum, it's far often sincerely a way of handling the extreme sensory and social stimulation that eye touch can convey.

Chapter 4: Not Smiling When You Smile At Them

Autistic humans regularly warfare with facial reputation, so in case you smile at them, they will not understand a way to answer. It isn't because of the fact they don't need to smile lower back or don't which encompass you; as a substitute, it's far because they will no longer be capable of decipher the social cues related to a smile. It is crucial to bear in mind that autistic human beings have a unique way of interpreting social cues and frequently depend on verbal communique in location of non-verbal communication which encompass facial expressions. As a stop end result, they'll now not be able to recognize the meaning of a smile or might not revel in comfortable in responding to it.

Additionally, autistic people also can have hassle information and interpreting the reactions of others, so they'll be uncertain of the manner to reply to a grin. It is crucial to be touchy to the truth that autistic humans may not continuously recognize or respond to facial expressions. Instead of watching for a smile in response on your smile, it is crucial to well known the man or woman's specific manner of expressing themselves. Communicating with terms, providing extraordinary reinforcement, and developing a solid and supportive environment can help autistic humans experience greater snug in responding for your smile.

Moreover, some autistic human beings can also moreover revel in extra snug if you offer verbal cues which encompass "I am smiling at you" or "I am glad to appearance you." Overall, it's miles crucial to take into account that autistic humans have a one of a type manner of interpreting and responding to social cues. The remarkable manner to talk with autistic human beings is to be affected individual, information, and use verbal conversation as opposed to counting on non-verbal communique which includes facial expressions.

GETTING VERY UPSET IF THEY DO NOT LIKE A
CERTAIN TASTE, SMELL OR SOUND.

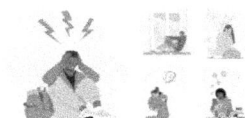

Autistic human beings can also experience
heightened sensitivity to positive tastes,
smells, and sounds. This can result in
immoderate misery if they may be exposed to
3 factor they find out ugly. The response to
tremendous tastes, smells, and sounds may
be so strong that it may reason an autistic
person to emerge as overwhelmed, agitated,
or even competitive. This form of reaction is
known as sensory overload. It can manifest at
the same time as an autistic person is
exposed to an excessive amount of sensory
enter proper now, or even as they are
uncovered to a stimulus this is specifically
unpleasant for them. The depth of the
reaction can variety from man or woman to

individual. Some can also additionally enjoy a slight soreness at the same time as others may also moreover grow to be especially distressed.

It is crucial to keep in thoughts that this response isn't always voluntary; it's miles an involuntary reaction to stimuli. In order to help an autistic character who's experiencing sensory overload, it's far critical to provide a stable, quiet, and snug surroundings. If feasible, remove the stimuli that is inflicting the misery. This can be a noisy sound, a robust fragrance, or a outstanding taste. If casting off the stimulus isn't feasible, then try to lessen the intensity of the stimulus. For example, if the individual is reacting to a noisy noise, use noise-cancelling headphones to reduce the sound. It is also vital to provide the man or woman with emotional assist.

Acknowledge their feelings and provide reassurance that they're steady. It also can assist to have a routine and offer shape and predictability to the environment. This will assist the individual experience greater stable and on pinnacle of factors. Finally, it is critical to remember that anybody is particular and what works for one person won't art work for each other. It is vital to be affected individual and flexible even as trying to help an autistic individual who's experiencing sensory overload.

REPETITIVE MOVEMENTS

Autistic human beings often show repetitive movements which incorporates hand flapping, rocking, spinning, and head banging. These behaviors are called stereotypic moves, and they arise for the duration of the autism spectrum. The unique motive of these repetitive movements is not appeared, but they are perception to be a stop give up end result of sensory issues. People with autism frequently struggle with sensory processing, and the repetitive movements are believed to be a way of supporting them cope with this problem.

This is supported with the aid of using the reality that these behaviors frequently lower whilst someone is given sensory enter this is calming or interesting. The repetitive movements moreover can be seen as a manner of self-stimulating, or providing a calming impact on the individual. Research has established that the ones behaviors are calming for autistic people, and might moreover be beneficial in helping them address tension and pressure. It is essential to be conscious that the ones repetitive movements aren't constantly complicated or risky. They may be a everyday a part of an autistic man or woman's existence, and need to be visible as a legitimate form of verbal exchange and self-expression.

Chapter 5: Abilities In Autism

Attention to element.

Autistic humans often monitor a outstanding capability to pay attention to information. This heightened hobby to element is a feature usually associated with autism and might seem in numerous ways. In this discussion, we can find out how autistic sufferers pay attention to data and the capability blessings and demanding situations associated with this cognitive trait.

One of the reasons autistic human beings excel in taking note of statistics is their specific cognitive processing fashion. Many autistic human beings own a cognitive profile that emphasizes close by processing over global processing. Local processing refers to a focal point on particular data and person factors of a state of affairs or mission, while worldwide processing consists of perceiving the overall context or massive picture. Autistic human beings normally generally tend to manifestly gravitate within the course of nearby processing, letting them take a look at and look at complex information that may work disregarded through others.

This interest to element often manifests specially regions of interest or expertise. Autistic humans can also show an extreme fascination with particular subjects, objects, or styles. This deep attention lets in them to immerse themselves in their pursuits and expand an notable stage of know-how or capability in the ones areas. This excessive focus and hobby to element can make a contribution to incredible records in fields in conjunction with mathematics, artwork, music, pc generation, or distinct specialized domain names.

Autistic people' attention to detail moreover may be decided in their eager assertion competencies. They might also additionally furthermore phrase patterns, inconsistencies, or minute adjustments in their environment that others might probably forget about. This heightened perceptual awareness can be precious in fields that require attention to detail, such as clinical research, engineering, or extraordinary manage. Autistic humans might also moreover furthermore excel in roles that name for precision and accuracy because of their capability to pick up on diffused nuances.

Furthermore, their hobby to element can increase to language and conversation. Some autistic humans display off a incredible memory for statistics, dates, or unique information associated with their pursuits. They might also additionally additionally show an acute experience of grammar, vocabulary, or linguistic styles. This interest to linguistic facts can bring about excellent language competencies and abilties, collectively with superior reading or writing capabilities.

While the ability to take note of records must have massive advantages, there are also ability challenges related to this cognitive trait. Autistic human beings can also grow to be beaten with the useful resource of sensory input because of their heightened sensitivity to info. They can also enjoy sensory overload in environments with immoderate noise, exquisite lighting, sturdy smells, or uncomfortable textures. Sensory overload can negatively effect their functionality to concentrate and method information.

Additionally, a hyperfocus on data can also lead to troubles in moving hobby or adapting to adjustments. Autistic humans may additionally moreover struggle with transitions, interruptions, or unexpected adjustments to their workout routines or responsibilities. This tension in interest can impact their flexibility and flexibility in fine conditions.

The interest to element exhibited thru autistic people moreover will growth issues regarding the wider cognitive profile. While they excel in unique regions, they'll face demanding conditions in other additives of cognitive functioning, which consist of precis reasoning, authorities skills, or social cognition. It is vital to apprehend that the eye to detail is absolutely one component in their cognitive abilties and need to be considered inside the context of the person's popular strengths and disturbing conditions.

Understanding and harnessing the attention to element in autistic human beings can be useful in severa processes. Educators can tailor instructional strategies to capitalize on their strengths and offer possibilities for deep exploration of specific subjects. Employers can create paintings environments that fee and leverage their interest to element, offering responsibilities that align with their exceptional observational abilties.

By recognizing and supporting their skills, we are capable of empower autistic human beings to thrive in areas wherein their interest to detail have to make a sizeable tremendous impact.

In give up, autistic people frequently very own a terrific capacity to be aware of statistics. This cognitive trait, associated with their precise cognitive processing style and immoderate cognizance, can make a contribution to know-how in specific domains and exquisite observational competencies. While there are functionality demanding situations associated with this cognitive trait, spotting and harnessing the attention to element can empower autistic human beings to excel in regions that align with their strengths and offer them with opportunities to make contributions their specific views and competencies to numerous fields.

Here are a few methods autistic sufferers can cultivate their interest to info:

Identify regions of hobby: Encourage the autistic person to find out and end up aware about topics or sports activities that virtually seize their interest and hobby. Supporting their passions can fuel their motivation and engagement, essential to progressed hobby to info within the ones unique areas.

Provide established environments: Establishing exercises and presenting a set up surroundings can assist autistic human beings preserve interest and interest to information. Clear schedules, visible helps, and predictable workouts can lessen tension and distractions, letting them deliver hobby to precise responsibilities or activities.

Break obligations into smaller steps: Complex responsibilities may be overwhelming, making it tough for autistic people to be privy to the essential info. Breaking responsibilities into smaller, functionality steps permits them interest on one factor at a time, making it less tough to approach and attend to information along the way.

Use visible supports: Visual aids, which embody visible schedules, checklists, or diagrams, can help in directing hobby to information. Visual representations provide concrete and organized facts, making it much less difficult for autistic individuals to approach and remember data.

Utilize sensory allows: Sensory sensitivities can every so often intrude with interest.

Providing sensory helps, along side noise-canceling headphones, fidget toys, or cushty seating, can help adjust sensory input and decorate reputation at the undertaking reachable.

Break down statistics visually: Presenting facts visually, via graphs, charts, or diagrams, can enhance facts and attention to facts for autistic individuals. Visual representations frequently offer a clearer and further organized depiction of facts, taking into consideration better comprehension and assessment of information.

Incorporate arms-on sports activities: Engaging in hands-on sports activities can promote interest to records. Encourage the usage of manipulatives, puzzles, or interactive substances that require statement and manipulation of unique factors.

Provide specific commands and feedback: Clear and precise instructions assist autistic human beings understand what is anticipated and direct their attention to particular records. Providing advantageous feedback and reinforcement for getting to facts also can encourage and beautify this conduct.

Practice mindfulness techniques: Teaching mindfulness techniques, together with deep respiration physical video video games or sensory grounding techniques, can assist autistic human beings enlarge attention and modify hobby. Mindfulness can promote a present-centered awareness that enhances interest to records inside the straight away surroundings.

Collaborate with specialists: Working with experts, together with occupational therapists or conduct analysts, can provide individualized strategies and interventions to help interest to records. These experts can boom customized plans and techniques tailor-made to the precise needs and strengths of the autistic character.

Chapter 6: Strong Memory

Autistic humans often show off a strong memory in diverse domain names, showcasing superb hold in mind abilities in particular regions of hobby. This cognitive energy can seem in wonderful methods and has been a subject of hobby in autism research. In this discussion, we are capable of discover the elements contributing to the robust reminiscence decided in a few autistic patients, the capacity blessings and traumatic conditions related to this trait, and techniques to guide and harness their reminiscence abilties.

Attention to Detail and Perceptual Strengths:

Autistic humans' hobby to element and perceptual strengths play a massive role of their sturdy memory. They frequently display off an excessive focus on precise statistics, styles, or gadgets, allowing them to have a have a look at and encode records in a significantly centered way. This level of hobby enhances their capacity to bear in mind and don't forget particular records as it should be.

Sensory-Based Memory:

Autistic individuals might also personal a sensory-based totally genuinely reminiscence, which incorporates encoding and retrieving statistics through sensory stimuli. They may have bright sensory reminiscences, associating specific data with sensory critiques which encompass attractions, sounds, smells, or textures. This sensory-based absolutely reminiscence lets in them to keep in mind sports activities or facts extra effectively even as associated with terrific sensory cues.

Pattern Recognition:

Many autistic human beings excel at pattern recognition, perceiving and identifying underlying patterns in statistics or conditions. This functionality contributes to their robust memory with the useful resource of letting them understand and keep in mind sequences, relationships, or institutions among one in all a type factors. Their sample-popularity abilties allow them to maintain and retrieve facts based on its context inner a bigger pattern or shape.

Systemizing Tendency:

Autistic human beings often show off a sturdy systemizing tendency, characterised via a force to apprehend and set up statistics into set up structures. This tendency may additionally enhance their reminiscence with the aid of manner of facilitating the organization and categorization of statistics, allowing efficient retrieval and bear in mind. Creating intellectual frameworks or categorizing records into logical structures lets in them to access saved information more truly.

Special Interests and Hyperfocus:

Autistic people often amplify severe unique hobbies in particular topics or subjects. Their passion and hyperfocus on those pastimes frequently purpose remarkable exploration and deep know-how acquisition. This focused engagement offers possibilities for repeated exposure and consolidation of information, leading to more suitable memory of their areas of hobby.

Rote Memory:

Some autistic humans show off a robust rote reminiscence, which includes the functionality to memorize and keep in thoughts data verbatim. They may also have an remarkable ability to keep actual facts, which incorporates numbers, dates, or unique data from books, movies, or conversations. This rote memory can contribute to their fantastic do not forget capabilities, especially in domain names that require particular facts retention.

Benefits of Strong Memory in Autism:

The strong reminiscence determined in autistic individuals can yield severa benefits:

a. Enhanced Learning: Their capability to keep and do not forget facts in element can facilitate powerful mastering, specifically in topics aligned with their interests. Autistic people can regularly take in and maintain large portions of records, allowing them to turn out to be experts of their decided on fields.

b. Academic Success: Their sturdy reminiscence can make contributions to academic success, as they may keep in mind data, formulation, or thoughts with precision. This strength may be notable in topics which includes mathematics, technological knowledge, facts, or language, wherein correct endure in mind and retention are important.

c. Attention to Detail: The robust reminiscence helps their interest to element, allowing them to word and bear in mind subtle nuances or patterns that others can also overlook about approximately. This hobby to element can be useful in severa professions, including studies, extraordinary control, or innovative endeavors.

d. Language and Communication Skills: Autistic human beings with robust memory frequently display advanced vocabulary, grammar, and language skills. They can keep in mind and utilize phrases and phrases successfully, contributing to their expressive and receptive language abilties.

e. Problem Solving and Logical Thinking: The functionality to recall and analyze statistics in detail can enhance their hassle-solving capabilities. Autistic people may additionally moreover excel in responsibilities requiring logical thinking, as they could preserve in mind and examine applicable information to make bigger solutions or make connections among apparently unrelated requirements.

Challenges Associated with Strong Memory in Autism:

While a sturdy reminiscence can offer blessings, it may moreover present disturbing situations for autistic human beings:

a. Selective Attention: Focusing on specific details or information can motive troubles in attending to broader contexts or filtering out irrelevant facts. Autistic human beings may also battle to prioritize and selectively attend to essential records while being inundated with numerous information.

b. Overwhelm and Sensory Overload: The excessive sensory and perceptual opinions associated with their reminiscence can lead to sensory overwhelm and sensory overload. Processing and recalling sensory statistics can be difficult, particularly in environments with immoderate sensory stimuli.

c. Contextual Understanding: While autistic human beings might also moreover excel in recalling precise records, they may war with knowledge the wider context or applying statistics flexibly. Difficulties in generalization and summary reasoning may additionally moreover restrict the switch in their memory abilities in some unspecified time in the future of specific contexts or domains.

d. Obsessive Thinking: Strong memory mixed with excessive pastimes or fixations can bring about obsessive thinking styles. Autistic humans may additionally moreover locate it tough to shift their interest an extended manner from their specific areas of interest, proscribing their recognition on considered one of a type essential elements of lifestyles.

Supporting and Harnessing Memory Abilities in Autism:

To resource and harness the memory abilities of autistic human beings, the following techniques may be implemented:

a. Visual Supports: Utilize visual aids, which incorporates seen schedules, photo organizers, or mind maps, to decorate business enterprise, retrieval, and keep in mind of statistics.

b. Structured Learning Environments: Establish installed and predictable learning environments to offer clarity and decrease distractions, allowing better consciousness and interest to data.

c. Multisensory Approaches: Incorporate multisensory techniques to facilitate memory encoding and retrieval. Combining visible, auditory, and tactile cues can decorate the connections among statistics and sensory reviews.

d. Mnemonic Techniques: Teach mnemonic techniques, which include acronyms, visualization, or rhythmic patterns, to useful resource reminiscence retention and recollect. These strategies can help in remembering complicated facts or sequences.

e. Chunking and Sequencing: Break down facts into smaller chunks or sequences to facilitate memory encoding and retrieval. Presenting facts in a installed and prepared way promotes green undergo in mind.

f. Contextualization: Help autistic human beings apprehend the context and application of facts by using manner of providing actual-life examples, practical demonstrations, or hands-on evaluations. Linking facts to real-international conditions can beautify comprehension and retention.

g. Support Transitions: Offer resource within the route of transitions among responsibilities or sports activities to lessen disruption to their reminiscence strategies. Provide increase be conscious and visual cues to help them mentally shift from one recognition of interest to another.

h. Individualized Approaches: Recognize the uniqueness of every individual's reminiscence skills and tailor strategies to their unique strengths and demanding conditions. Collaborate with the character, their aid network, and specialists to increase personalized techniques that optimize their memory functionality.

Chapter 7: Logical Thinking

Logical thinking is a cognitive technique that consists of reasoning, analyzing records, and drawing conclusions based on proof and guidelines. It is the capability to method troubles, conditions, and desire-making in a established, systematic, and rational manner. Logical thinking is characterised with the aid of manner of an emphasis on coherence, consistency, and logical frameworks, permitting people to make sound judgments and arrive at nicely-founded conclusions.

At its middle, logical wondering is ready the usage of logical mind and guidelines to technique information and attain logical conclusions. It includes the following key additives:

Reasoning: Logical wondering calls for the capability to engage in reasoning, which incorporates making inferences, deducing relationships, and drawing conclusions based totally on proof and logical regulations. Reasoning lets in human beings to evaluate information, find out connections, and examine relationships among mind or elements.

Analysis: Logical thinking involves breaking down complex information or problems into smaller, greater viable components. Through evaluation, people can test the information, pick out out patterns, and understand the underlying shape of the facts. This step-with the useful aid of-step evaluation enables a scientific and entire understanding of the facts.

Evidence-based Approach: Logical wondering emphasizes the reliance on proof and actual records. It calls for people to accumulate relevant statistics, look into its credibility and validity, and use it to help their reasoning and conclusions. By considering the proof, logical thinkers can keep away from biases and make more aim exams.

Rule-Based Thinking: Logical questioning regularly includes using guidelines or ideas to remedy problems or make picks. These regulations can be derived from various sources on the aspect of logical frameworks, installation theories, or empirical observations. Rule-based totally questioning gives a based technique to reasoning and allows people set up consistency and coherence in their thinking techniques.

Deductive and Inductive Reasoning: Logical questioning encompasses each deductive and inductive reasoning. Deductive reasoning includes drawing precise conclusions from famous mind or premises. Inductive reasoning, as an alternative, involves inferring famous ideas or conclusions primarily based mostly on particular observations or evidence. Both varieties of reasoning play a essential characteristic in logical questioning, permitting humans to make logical connections amongst thoughts and proof.

Pattern Recognition: Logical wondering often calls for people to understand and understand styles or regularities in facts. By detecting patterns, people must make predictions, find out relationships, and comply with logical reasoning to solve problems. Pattern recognition is an crucial talents that enables in organizing statistics and making informed judgments.

Critical Thinking: Logical thinking is carefully intertwined with critical questioning. Critical questioning includes comparing arguments, questioning assumptions, and difficult the validity of data. It encourages humans to take into account opportunity views, weigh proof, and investigate the logical coherence of arguments. Critical wondering enhances logical wondering with the useful aid of fostering a more thorough and rigorous assessment of data.

Benefits of Logical Thinking in Autism:

The logical thinking abilties exhibited with the resource of autistic human beings offer numerous advantages:

a. Problem-Solving Abilities: Autistic people often excel in trouble-solving due to their logical wondering skills. They can smash down complicated troubles into feasible factors, observe pointers and patterns, and systematically have a look at information to attain at powerful solutions.

b. Attention to Detail: Their eager interest to element permits them to identify nuances and subtleties that others can also pass over. This interest to element guarantees thorough assessment and allows them to do not forget all relevant elements of their selection-making.

c. Rule Adherence: Autistic individuals' inclination to comply with regulations and processes contributes to their capability to make sound judgments. They prioritize consistency and logical frameworks, which helps them arrive at reliable conclusions and make informed alternatives.

d. Accuracy and Precision: Autistic human beings' logical questioning often leads to accurate and specific assessments. They have the functionality to investigate information systematically, making sure that their conclusions are based mostly on strong evidence and logical reasoning.

e. Organizational Skills: The logical wondering abilities of autistic humans make a contribution to their robust organizational capabilities. They can create systems and systems to categorize and manage facts efficaciously, improving their functionality to stay organized and focused.

f. Attention to Patterns: Autistic people' tremendous pattern recognition talents allow them to select out underlying styles and relationships. This ability lets in them apprehend complex structures, anticipate effects, and make connections that others might not right away understand.

Challenges Associated with Logical Thinking in Autism:

While logical questioning is a energy for plenty autistic people, it can moreover gift challenges:

a. Rigidity in Thinking: Autistic individuals may additionally show off inflexible questioning patterns, that might limit their capability to take into account opportunity views or solutions. Their adherence to guidelines and structures also can hinder flexibility in hassle-fixing and choice-making.

b. Difficulty with Abstract Concepts: Some autistic humans may additionally battle with summary or hypothetical thinking. Logical questioning often includes the manipulation of summary ideas, which can be hard for folks that especially have interaction in concrete questioning.

c. Processing Overload: The interest to detail and focus on systematic processing can bring about facts overload. Autistic people can also emerge as beaten with the useful resource of immoderate info or conflict to prioritize and easy out data effectively.

d. Contextual Understanding: While logical wondering focuses on analyzing records and patterns, autistic human beings can also additionally battle with records the wider context of a state of affairs. They can also find out it difficult to apply logical reasoning to actual-worldwide situations that comprise complicated social or emotional dynamics.

e. Challenges in Collaborative Settings: Logical thinking in autistic human beings may be at odds with the social nature of collaborative environments. Their emphasis on guidelines and structures may also struggle with the ability and compromise required in organization settings, main to problems in collaborative hassle-solving.

Supporting and Nurturing Logical Thinking in Autism:

To useful resource and nurture the logical wondering skills of autistic people, the following techniques can be accomplished:

a. Providing Clear Instructions: Clear and concise commands help autistic humans apprehend expectations and interact in logical thinking tactics correctly. Avoiding ambiguous or vague language promotes readability and complements their capability to comply with logical steps.

b. Visual Supports: Utilizing visible aids, which includes seen schedules, flowcharts, or diagrams, can help autistic people in organizing their thoughts and visually representing logical strategies.

c. Teaching Problem-Solving Strategies: Introducing hassle-solving techniques, which includes breaking down complicated duties, identifying applicable information, and considering opportunity answers, can beautify their functionality to technique troubles logically.

d. Encouraging Flexibility: Balancing logical thinking with flexibility is essential. Encouraging autistic people to remember awesome perspectives, entertain possibility answers, and adapt their questioning to unique conditions promotes flexibility internal logical frameworks.

e. Providing Structured Environments: Establishing based totally environments that include steady exercises and smooth rules can assist the logical taking into consideration autistic people. Predictability and company assist create a foundation for logical assessment and choice-making.

f. Promoting Social Interactions: Encouraging social interactions and collaboration can help autistic people look at logical wondering capabilities in social contexts. Group problem-solving sports activities that emphasize teamwork and compromise can facilitate the improvement of collaborative thinking.

g. Emphasizing Real-World Applications: Linking logical questioning to actual-international packages lets in autistic people apprehend the sensible relevance of their competencies. Providing examples and possibilities to apply logical questioning in everyday situations fosters transferability and generalization.

Chapter 8: Intense Interest

Autistic humans often show off an severe hobby on unique topics, sports activities, or gadgets. This characteristic is generally referred to as "particular interests" or "hyperfocus." The excessive cognizance displayed through using autistic people will have every first-rate and tough additives. In this dialogue, we are able to explore the man or woman of immoderate interest in autism, its benefits, disturbing conditions, and techniques to assist people with this trait.

Nature of Intense Focus:

Intense interest refers back to the functionality of autistic individuals to pay interest deeply on precise topics or sports activities for prolonged durations. This reputation may also comprise a slim range of interests, which include trains, dinosaurs, or arithmetic, or it can encompass particular abilities, like drawing or programming. Autistic people can also display remarkable understanding, information, and willpower of their selected regions of hobby.

Benefits of Intense Focus:

Intense cognizance gives numerous benefits for autistic individuals:

a. Enhanced Knowledge and Expertise: Intense hobby allows people to boom large information and records of their areas of interest. They can also additionally moreover gather in-depth data, memorize complex records, and display a deep know-how in their decided on topics.

b. Motivation and Engagement: The severe recognition experienced with the useful resource of autistic human beings regularly results in immoderate stages of motivation and engagement. Their passionate interest in a particular subject matter or activity drives them to discover, have a study, and excel in their decided on domain.

c. Skill Development: Intense attention can bring about the improvement of top notch abilties. Autistic people may also commit big time and effort to exercise and refine their competencies, leading to extraordinary achievements of their targeted areas.

d. Sense of Identity and Purpose: Intense consciousness offers autistic individuals with a sense of identity and purpose. It allows them to cultivate a sturdy revel in of self and derive that means from their pursuits, contributing to their normal well-being and vanity.

Challenges of Intense Focus:

While excessive consciousness may be useful, it may furthermore present demanding situations:

a. Narrowed Focus: The extreme hobby of autistic humans frequently outcomes in a slender range of interests. They might also moreover warfare to have interaction in activities out of doors their centered areas, proscribing their publicity to diverse critiques.

b. Difficulty with Transitions: Shifting hobby from their excessive consciousness to different obligations or topics may be difficult for autistic humans. Abrupt transitions or interruptions also can purpose distress or frustration, as they prefer to maintain their hobby on their desired sports sports.

c. Social Isolation: Intense cognizance may bring about social isolation, as autistic individuals might also battle to hook up with others who do not percentage their particular hobbies. This isolation may have an impact on social interactions and restriction opportunities for diverse social connections.

d. Imbalance in Daily Life: The intense popularity of autistic human beings can once in a while disrupt daily workout routines and responsibilities. They also can prioritize their particular pastimes over essential responsibilities, fundamental to difficulties in handling time and duties.

Strategies to Support Intense Focus:

Supporting humans with immoderate reputation can help harness their strengths even as addressing functionality worrying situations:

a. Balancing Activities: Encourage a stability among targeted hobbies and different sports. Introduce new research and step by step expand their regions of interest to promote a broader range of engagement.

b. Time Management and Transitions: Teach techniques for handling time and transitioning among activities. Visual schedules, timers, and easy conversation about upcoming adjustments can help people in navigating transitions extra easily.

c. Integration of Interests: Explore processes to integrate centered pursuits into unique regions of lifestyles. For example, incorporating a special interest into college assignments or seeking out associated social possibilities can create connections and facilitate broader engagement.

d. Social Skills Development: Provide opportunities for social talents development and interaction with buddies who percentage comparable hobbies. This can help amplify social connections and decrease social isolation.

e. Building Flexibility: Gradually introduce flexibility and flexibility into their exercises. Encourage exploration of recent pursuits and sports whilst retaining guide for their contemporary focused interests.

f. Parent and Educator Collaboration: Collaboration among mother and father, educators, and therapists is important in understanding the individual's intense cognizance and developing suitable strategies to assist their learning and standard development.

Visual wondering

Autistic people often display off a completely particular cognitive fashion referred to as seen questioning. Visual wondering refers back to the capability to manner and recognize records essentially thru visible highbrow imagery in preference to depending totally on verbal or auditory processing.

This mode of questioning permits autistic people to understand, have a look at, and constitute the arena in seen styles, photographs, and spatial relationships. In this speak, we will find out the developments, strengths, and challenges related to visible questioning in autism.

Characteristics of Visual Thinking:

a. Mental Imagery: Autistic people who have interplay in visible wondering have a strong functionality to form colorful highbrow pix. They can create notable visible representations of gadgets, thoughts, and situations in their minds.

b. Visual Patterns and Relationships: Visual thinkers excel in recognizing and expertise styles, connections, and relationships among items or ideas. They can apprehend similarities, versions, and spatial arrangements by relying on seen cues and imagery.

c. Thinking in Pictures: Visual thinkers frequently device statistics within the shape of intellectual pix or visible representations. They might also moreover additionally mentally visualize ideas, activities, or commands, permitting them to draw near facts extra efficiently.

d. Visual Problem-Solving: Autistic individuals with visible thinking talents approach trouble-fixing duties with the aid of mentally manipulating seen photos. They can visualize super situations, test ability solutions, and anticipate consequences, helping in progressive problem-fixing.

e. Spatial Awareness: Visual thinkers commonly commonly generally tend to have robust spatial cognizance and visualization skills. They can mentally map and navigate physical areas, preserve in thoughts seen details of their surroundings, and apprehend spatial relationships because it must be.

Strengths of Visual Thinking:

a. Visual Memory: Autistic individuals with visible questioning frequently own tremendous visual memory. They can bear in thoughts and hold visible statistics with amazing accuracy, which may be first rate in obligations which includes memorization, consider, and reputation.

b. Detail-Oriented Analysis: Visual thinkers have a eager eye for element. They excel at noticing and reading visible data that others would possibly probably neglect. This interest to element may be valuable in fields together with artwork, design, and medical announcement.

c. Visual Problem-Solving: Visual thinking lets in autistic people to approach problem-solving responsibilities from precise views. Their capability to mentally control seen pictures and understand patterns can purpose present day solutions and methods.

d. Visual Creativity: Visual thinkers often display off innovative competencies through visible arts, design, and special visually-oriented disciplines. They can generate precise and resourceful mind thru manner of drawing on their wealthy visible imagery.

Challenges of Visual Thinking:

a. Language-Based Tasks: Visual thinkers may also moreover war with language-based totally duties that rely closely on verbal or auditory processing. This can consist of worrying situations in records and expressing summary requirements, following complex verbal instructions, or wearing out prolonged verbal discussions.

b. Communication Differences: Autistic human beings with visible wondering can also face difficulties in successfully speakme their thoughts and mind, especially in situations wherein verbal communique is the primary mode. They might also moreover moreover depend upon visible aids, gestures, or opportunity communique strategies to bridge the gap.

c. Processing Overload: In environments with immoderate visible stimuli, visible thinkers may additionally experience sensory overload. They can also furthermore end up beaten via the usage of the abundance of visible records, fundamental to problems in focusing or filtering out beside the aspect statistics.

Strategies to Support Visual Thinking:

a. Visual Supports: Provide visual aids, collectively with charts, diagrams, or written commands, to help individuals with visible questioning understand and bear in mind data. Visual enables can beautify comprehension, industrial agency corporation, and verbal exchange.

Chapter 9: Special Pursuits

Special interests are a incredible function in plenty of autistic people. A unique interest, additionally referred to as a "targeted interest" or "obsession," refers to an intense and enduring fascination with a specific challenge be counted, hassle, or hobby. Autistic human beings regularly reveal a passionate strength of will to their particular pastimes, making an funding great time and power into exploring, analyzing, and appealing with them. In this communicate, we are able to discover the individual of unique interests, their benefits, traumatic conditions, and strategies for supporting people with this element of autism.

Nature of Special Interests:

a. Intensity and Focus: Special interests in autistic people are characterized by way of the usage of a high degree of depth and interest. They frequently grow to be deeply engrossed in their decided on difficulty depend, dedicating substantial time and interest to getting to know and exploring every factor of it.

b. Narrow Range of Interests: Special interests will be predisposed to be specific and narrow in scope. Autistic humans may additionally expand excessive passions for subjects like dinosaurs, trains, astronomy, laptop programming, or specific intervals of statistics.

c. Expertise and Knowledge: Engaging especially interests allows human beings to accumulate enormous know-how and knowledge in their selected region. They frequently reveal a splendid degree of know-how and may don't forget complicated data, data, and figures related to their hobby.

d. Emotional Investment: Special pursuits are not surely intellectual pursuits however additionally incorporate a deep emotional investment. Autistic people may also moreover experience a sturdy emotional connection, delight, and success whilst attractive with their unique interest.

Benefits of Special Interests:

a. Motivation and Engagement: Special pursuits offer autistic human beings with a strong supply of motivation and engagement. They can characteristic a effective the usage of pressure, promoting gaining knowledge of, exploration, and personal increase.

b. Skill Development: Immersion in a totally unique interest frequently ends within the improvement of notable competencies. Autistic human beings may additionally additionally moreover acquire specialised understanding, technical know-how, and specific talents associated with their interest.

c. Sense of Identity: Special pastimes contribute to the formation of a experience of identification for autistic human beings. They provide a supply of pride, vanity, and a feel of belonging, permitting humans to outline themselves via their passions.

d. Coping Mechanism: Special pastimes can feature a valuable coping mechanism for autistic individuals. They provide a predictable and established outlet for pressure treatment, emotional law, and a enjoy of manage in a now and again overwhelming global.

Challenges of Special Interests:

a. Narrow Focus and Limited Interests: Special interests can result in a narrowed attention, limiting the individual's engagement in other areas of existence. This may also moreover impact social interactions, educational pursuits, or the improvement of a properly-rounded skills set.

b. Difficulty with Transitions: Shifting interest from the special hobby to distinct responsibilities or sports may be difficult for autistic human beings. Abrupt transitions or interruptions may additionally moreover moreover reason misery or frustration, as they prefer to keep their reputation on their favored hobby.

c. Social Isolation: The slim and excessive recognition on a completely precise hobby can now and again bring about social isolation. Autistic human beings might also battle to connect to friends who do no longer share their particular hobby, making it hard to initiate or maintain social interactions.

d. Imbalance in Daily Life: An overwhelming preoccupation with a completely unique interest may additionally disrupt day by day exercises and responsibilities. Individuals can also prioritize their hobby over critical duties, main to issues in coping with time, self-care, or exceptional obligations.

Strategies to Support Special Interests:

a. Encouragement and Validation: Acknowledge the importance and value of the particular interest. Provide effective reinforcement, encouragement, and validation, expressing interest in the person's know-how, accomplishments, and electricity of mind.

b. Integration into Learning: Incorporate the particular hobby into academic sports activities and assignments. This integration can decorate motivation, engagement, and the purchase of broader competencies and know-how.

c. Facilitating Social Connections: Help individuals with particular hobbies connect to like-minded friends or communities who percentage their passion. This can create opportunities for social interplay, collaboration, and the sharing of critiques and information.

d. Balancing Activities: Encourage a stability most of the precise interest and different factors of lifestyles. Introduce new reviews, pastimes, or topics little by little, deliberating a broader variety of engagement and know-how development.

e. Flexibility and Transitions: Support the improvement of pliability and coping techniques for transitioning a number of the particular hobby and one in all a type sports.

Use visible schedules, timers, or verbal reminders to assist individuals manage transitions extra effortlessly.

f. Collaboration and Communication: Foster open conversation and collaboration a few of the man or woman, circle of relatives members, educators, and therapists. This collaboration can bring about a higher records of the unique interest, its impact, and the development of supportive strategies.

Honesty and directness

Autistic people are regularly seemed for his or her directness and honesty in conversation. This detail of their communication fashion may be attributed to pleasant dispositions normally placed in autism. In this discussion, we are able to explore why autistic humans have a tendency to be direct and honest and the way the ones dispositions seem of their conversation.

Cognitive Style:

Autistic human beings frequently have a concrete and literal wondering fashion. They have a propensity to interpret records and communicate in a honest manner, focusing at the literal that means of terms and phrases. This cognitive style contributes to their directness in communique, as they particular themselves in reality with out relying on subtle or indirect language.

Difficulty with Social Nuances:

Autistic humans can also battle with social nuances and nonverbal conversation cues, together with sarcasm, irony, or hidden meanings. As a end end result, they will be much more likely to talk in an immediate and literal manner, declaring their mind and observations with out embellishment or hidden agendas.

Preference for Clarity and Precision:

Autistic people regularly rate readability and precision in communique. They also can have a strong choice to convey information because it should be and keep away from confusion or ambiguity. This preference for clear and concise conversation leads them to express themselves right now and without a doubt.

Sensory Sensitivities:

Many autistic individuals have sensory sensitivities which can impact their communication. They may additionally discover it difficult to easy out outside stimuli and recognition mostly on the verbal exchange to hand. This sensory overload can bring about a greater trustworthy and centered verbal exchange fashion, as they're attempting to preserve their message correctly.

Honesty as a Core Value:

Autistic individuals regularly have a robust experience of honesty as a center cost. They typically tend to stick to tips and thoughts, and lying or being deceptive may match toward their moral compass. As a result, they may be much more likely to explicit their thoughts and observations surely and in reality.

Challenges in Social Masking:

Social protecting refers to the act of concealing one's autistic trends at the way to fit into social norms. While a few autistic people interact in protecting to diverse stages, it may be mentally and emotionally difficult. When they'll be unable to hold social overlaying, their natural directness and honesty can also turn out to be extra apparent in their communication.

It is essential to notice that while directness and honesty are normally related to autistic humans, no longer every autistic person famous the ones tendencies to the equal degree. Communication styles can in spite of the reality that range amongst autistic people primarily based totally on their individual personalities, reviews, and levels of help.

Benefits of Direct and Honest Communication:

Clarity and Transparency: Direct verbal exchange can reduce misunderstandings and sell clean and particular exchanges of records.

Trust and Authenticity: Autistic humans' honesty fosters accept as true with and authenticity in their relationships, as they're often perceived as dependable and real communicators.

Efficiency in Communication: Their truthful technique can result in more inexperienced conversations, as they will be predisposed to popularity on the crucial statistics and avoid useless complexities.

Supporting Autistic Individuals in Communication:

Encourage Active Listening: Active listening skills can help each autistic people and their communication partners to understand and reply correctly to every different's perspectives.

Provide Feedback and Guidance: Offer constructive feedback and steerage to help autistic individuals navigate social nuances and understand the effect of their communique fashion in amazing contexts.

Promote Social Skills Development: Support the improvement of social abilities through primarily based social abilities schooling programs or remedy, in which people can learn how to apprehend and reply efficaciously to social cues and nonverbal verbal exchange.

Chapter 10: Sensory Sensitivity

Sensory sensitivity, moreover called sensory processing troubles or sensory sensitivities, is a commonplace feature placed in lots of autistic humans. It refers to ordinary responses to sensory stimuli, in which people can also have heightened or decreased sensitivity to sensory records from the environment or their very very personal our our bodies. In this communicate, we are capable of explore sensory sensitivity in autistic people, its impact on daily life, and strategies for coping with and supporting people who revel in sensory sensitivities.

Types of Sensory Sensitivities:

a. Hyper-Sensitivity: Hyper-sensitivity refers to heightened sensitivity to sensory enter. Autistic folks who experience hyper-sensitivity may additionally additionally locate effective sounds, elements of interest, textures, tastes, or smells overwhelming or painful. They may additionally have a decrease threshold for sensory stimulation and can end up without problems overstimulated.

b.   Hypo-Sensitivity: Hypo-sensitivity, however, refers to reduced sensitivity to sensory enter. Autistic folks that revel in hypo-sensitivity may additionally additionally have a higher threshold for sensory stimulation and may are looking for out excessive sensory testimonies. They may additionally additionally require more potent or extra common sensory enter to test in sensations.

Impact on Daily Life:

Sensory sensitivities can notably effect an autistic character's each day life in severa tactics:

a. Sensory Overload: Overstimulation from sensory input can reason sensory overload, inflicting pressure, anxiety, or meltdowns. Common triggers embody loud noises, colourful lighting, crowded environments, or pleasant textures.

b. Sensory Avoidance: Individuals with sensory sensitivities can also actively avoid or are in search of to lessen publicity to positive sensory stimuli which might be uncomfortable or overwhelming to them. This can affect their participation in every day sports, social interactions, and get admission to to numerous environments.

c. Impact on Functioning: Sensory sensitivities can intrude with an character's functionality to pay attention, research, or engage in duties. For example, sensitivity to history noise in a observe room may additionally additionally make it tough for them to attention on schooling.

d. Emotional Regulation: Sensory sensitivities can impact emotional law. Overwhelming sensory reviews may additionally additionally cause emotions of frustration, irritability, or tension, probably predominant to emotional outbursts or shutdowns.

Common Sensory Sensitivities:

Autistic people might also additionally moreover display off sensitivities in unique sensory domains:

a. Auditory Sensitivities: Certain sounds, together with loud noises, precise frequencies, or statistics noise, can be specially distressing or overwhelming.

b. Visual Sensitivities: Bright lighting, fluorescent lighting fixtures, or extreme visual patterns may additionally moreover additionally purpose ache or sensory overload.

c. Tactile Sensitivities: Some people can also have heightened sensitivity to touch, textures, or apparel, locating certain fabric, tags, or specific sensations uncomfortable or painful.

d. Gustatory and Olfactory Sensitivities: Certain tastes or smells may be overwhelming or aversive, predominant to meals aversions or ache in positive environments.

e. Proprioceptive and Vestibular Sensitivities: Sensitivities to frame function, motion, or stability can effect an man or woman's functionality to interact in sports activities activities that include coordination, spatial attention, or physical contact.

Strategies for Managing Sensory Sensitivities:

a. Environmental Modifications: Create a sensory-satisfactory environment thru lowering useless stimuli, providing a quiet region, the use of clean lighting fixtures, or allowing the man or woman to apply headphones or shades as wanted.

b. Sensory Diet: Develop a sensory food plan, which incorporates sports that help adjust sensory input, which includes deep pressure sports sports, fidget system, or sensory breaks.

c. Sensory Accommodations: Advocate for sensory hotels in academic or artwork settings, along with preferential seating, use of noise-cancelling headphones, or get admission to to sensory-nice areas.

d. Communication and Self-Advocacy: Encourage people to speak their sensory desires and possibilities to others. This can embody expressing ache or requesting modifications in sensory environments.

e. Occupational Therapy: Engage in occupational treatment to extend strategies and coping mechanisms to govern sensory sensitivities successfully.

f. Gradual Exposure and Desensitization: Introduce sensory stimuli regularly and in a controlled manner, permitting the person to turn out to be extra snug and desensitized over the years.

g. Individualized Approaches: Recognize that sensory sensitivities are specific to every character. Collaborate with the person to increase customized techniques that deal with their precise sensitivities and desires.

Logical reasoning

Logical reasoning refers to the machine of the usage of rational and systematic questioning to attain at conclusions or make picks primarily based mostly on logical principles and proof. It involves the functionality to research data, understand patterns, relationships, and connections, and draw logical inferences or deductions. Logical reasoning is an vital cognitive skill that permits humans to assume seriously, clear up problems, and make sound judgments.

The key additives of logical reasoning encompass:

Premises: Logical reasoning begins offevolved with a difficult and speedy of premises or statements that provide the idea for the reasoning process. These premises can be records, observations, assumptions, or installation standards.

Rules of Logic: Logical reasoning follows unique rules and standards of commonplace feel, together with deductive or inductive reasoning, to derive legitimate conclusions from the given premises. These pointers assist make certain that the reasoning approach is logical, ordinary, and reliable.

Analysis: Logical reasoning involves studying the premises and breaking them down into smaller additives to apprehend their that means, implications, and relationships. This evaluation lets in recognize relevant records, styles, and logical connections amongst terrific factors.

Inferences: Based on the assessment of the premises, logical reasoning permits human beings to draw inferences or logical conclusions. Inferences are logical deductions or conclusions that have a look at from the given premises or evidence. They are based totally totally on the software of logical recommendations and mind to the analyzed information.

Problem-Solving: Logical reasoning plays a essential position in trouble-fixing. It allows humans to evaluate and take a look at special alternatives or solutions, weigh the evidence and capacity outcomes, and make informed picks based totally absolutely totally on logical evaluation.

Critical Thinking: Logical reasoning is cautiously linked to vital wondering, which includes comparing records, thinking assumptions, thinking about possibility views, and making reasoned judgments. Critical thinking allows people decide the validity and reliability of arguments, apprehend logical fallacies, and avoid errors in reasoning.

Pattern Recognition: Logical reasoning regularly includes recognizing patterns, relationships, and inclinations in records or records. This capability to turn out to be aware of and apprehend styles permits individuals to make generalizations, predictions, or draw conclusions based totally on determined regularities.

Logical reasoning has numerous realistic packages in various domain names, which includes generation, mathematics, philosophy, law, pc programming, and everyday trouble-fixing. It enables human beings study complex conditions, examine arguments, recognize cause-and-effect relationships, and make logical and informed picks.

In educational settings, logical reasoning is regularly emphasized as a important skills for instructional achievement. It is nurtured through sports activities which includes puzzles, logical reasoning video video games, crucial wondering sporting activities, and the look at of logical thoughts and strategies.

Chapter 11: Unique Attitude

Autistic people can exhibit specific views due to the variations in how their brains gadget data and understand the arena. Autism is a neurodevelopmental scenario that influences social interaction, verbal exchange, and conduct. While every autistic man or woman is unique and memories the arena of their private manner, there are some commonplace tendencies that may make contributions to their specific views:

Sensory processing: Many autistic human beings have variations in sensory processing, which can result in heightened or dwindled sensitivity to sensory stimuli. They may additionally additionally phrase facts or styles that others would likely overlook and enjoy the arena in a greater excessive or precise manner.

Attention to detail: Autistic humans frequently have a sturdy hobby to detail and can focus on unique elements in their surroundings or responsibilities. This hobby to detail can cause specific observations and perspectives that others might not have taken into consideration.

Non-linear wondering: Autistic thinking styles can be non-linear, that means they may make connections and institutions that are not right now obvious to others. This can result in unique and innovative views on various topics.

Systemizing tendency: Many autistic humans have a herbal inclination within the path of systemizing, which includes knowledge and growing structures, patterns, or policies. This tendency can bring about unique processes of categorizing facts or facts complicated principles.

Intense pastimes: Autistic human beings frequently make bigger intense pastimes in specific subjects, every so often called "unique interests." They may also moreover acquire big expertise approximately the ones topics and method them from a totally unique attitude that others may not percentage.

Enhanced visual thinking: Some autistic individuals have robust visible questioning abilities, which could make contributions to unique perspectives. They might imagine in pix and use seen representations to recognize and explicit their mind.

It's important to word that at the same time as autistic humans also can offer precise views, their research and viewpoints can variety broadly. It's usually excellent to pay attention to and recognize the man or woman's very very own mind and feelings, as they'll be the professionals on their personal reminiscences.

A specific thoughts-set refers to an person's first rate way of perceiving and understanding the area primarily based absolutely totally on their private opinions, developments, and ideals. It is stimulated through different factors consisting of cultural heritage, schooling, non-public information, and cognitive methods. Here are a few key elements to don't forget while discussing unique perspectives:

Subjectivity: Perspectives are inherently subjective, fashioned with the resource of the usage of an character's specific set of recollections, emotions, and values. No two human beings have exactly the same historical past or attitude, which ends up in severa perspectives.

Cultural range: Cultural backgrounds extensively have an effect on views. Different cultures have brilliant values, traditions, and ideals that form how humans recognize the arena. This variety gives richness and depth to our understanding of numerous subjects.

Personal tales: Our personal opinions form our perspectives. Each character has a very precise existence journey with encounters, disturbing situations, and triumphs that have an effect on how they recognize and interpret the sector round them. These reviews can provide smooth insights and alternative viewpoints.

Cognitive variations: Variances in cognitive strategies, inclusive of logical reasoning, creativity, reminiscence, or hobby, can result in severa views. Individuals can also approach issues or conditions in any other case primarily based absolutely totally on their cognitive strengths and weaknesses.

Alternative viewpoints: Unique perspectives venture prevailing norms, assumptions, and conventional interest. They offer clean insights, alternative solutions, and new processes of wondering. Embracing various views can foster innovation, creativity, and trouble-solving.

Empathy and facts: Recognizing and information specific views fosters empathy and enhances interpersonal relationships. It permits us to increase our horizons, recognize particular viewpoints, and growth a more complete know-how of complex troubles.

Multiple lenses: Approaching a subject from a couple of views can offer a greater holistic expertise. By thinking about numerous

141

viewpoints, we're able to gain a deeper belief into the nuances and complexities of a subject.

Overcoming biases: Embracing specific perspectives permits venture and overcome biases. It encourages crucial questioning and open-mindedness, considering a greater balanced and inclusive technique to choice-making and problem-fixing.

Importance in choice-making: Incorporating numerous views in choice-making strategies promotes fairness, inclusivity, and nicely-rounded results. It reduces the chance of overlooking essential elements or making biased judgments.

Bridge-constructing: Unique views can act as bridges among precise businesses, fostering speak, records, and cooperation. They can facilitate the exchange of thoughts and the combination of severa viewpoints, fundamental to more potent communities and businesses.

Here are some key elements of the particular views frequently exhibited with the aid of autistic people:

Attention to element: Many autistic people have a notable capability to be aware and recognition on information that others may additionally neglect about. This interest to detail can lead to particular observations and perspectives on diverse subjects. They may choose up on styles, inconsistencies, or intricacies that others might not correctly recognize.

Different sensory reviews: Sensory processing versions are not unusual amongst autistic human beings. They may additionally moreover experience sensory stimuli, which includes sounds, textures, tastes, or smells, greater intensely or otherwise in contrast to neurotypical human beings. This heightened or dwindled sensitivity can provide them with specific perspectives on their environment and the way they interact with it.

Non-linear questioning: Autistic thinking styles frequently show off a non-linear nature. They also can make connections and establishments that aren't proper now apparent to others. This non-linear wondering fashion can bring about unique and modern views on a huge form of topics, as they'll approach troubles or situations from unconventional angles.

Systemizing dispositions: Many autistic humans have a herbal inclination towards systemizing. They revel in growing and knowledge structures, patterns, or tips. This tendency can contribute to unique perspectives, as they may view and interpret information thru a scientific lens, noticing relationships and systems that others won't with out problems understand.

Intense pastimes and specialized information: Autistic people frequently broaden severe pastimes particularly subjects, sometimes called "specific hobbies." They dedicate significant effort and time to acquiring facts in the ones regions, becoming rather knowledgeable and obsessed on their selected subjects. This information can offer them with a very particular mind-set and intensity of know-how that others won't personal.

Enhanced visible thinking: Some autistic people display off robust visual wondering capabilities. They may think in photos and use visual representations to recognize and communicate their mind. This visible questioning fashion can offer specific views and progressive trouble-solving procedures, as they'll visualize standards or situations in strategies that alternate from verbal or linear questioning.

Emotional sensitivity: Autistic human beings also can have heightened emotional sensitivity, experiencing emotions intensely or in outstanding methods in assessment to neurotypical people. This emotional intensity can provide them with precise insights and perspectives on human studies, relationships, and societal dynamics.

It is crucial to go through in mind that those traits and perspectives can variety significantly amongst autistic people. Each character has their non-public precise combination of strengths, disturbing conditions, and views. Embracing and valuing the ones numerous views can foster understanding, popularity, and inclusivity in society.

Resilience and perseverance.

Resilience and perseverance are essential inclinations that permit human beings to overcome boundaries and thrive regardless of adversity. For autistic individuals, who navigate a global that might not continuously recognize or accommodate their particular needs, resilience and perseverance play a vital characteristic in their non-public increase and properly-being. This essay explores the factors that make a contribution to the resilience and perseverance of autistic human beings, highlighting their power, dedication, and capability to thrive in the face of disturbing conditions.

Self-Awareness and Self-Advocacy:

One crucial element of resilience in autistic people is the development of self-recognition. Autistic people often undergo a procedure of self-discovery, expertise their strengths, annoying conditions, and sensory sensitivities. This self-attention allows them to apprehend their very own dreams, set practical desires, and advocate for themselves successfully. By knowledge their particular traits and choices, they may talk their necessities to others, are searching for help whilst wanted, and actively take part in shaping their non-public lives.

Harnessing Special Interests and Strengths:

Many autistic people increase severe interests in unique subjects, commonly referred to as "unique interests." These pursuits can provide a deep sense of motivation, joy, and reason. Autistic people often personal top notch information and records in their regions of interest, leveraging their strengths to overcome demanding situations. Engaging in sports aligned with their passions lets in them to faucet into their ability, bolster their self-self guarantee, and discover success even amidst troubles.

Problem-Solving Skills and Alternative Thinking:

Autistic humans regularly show off unique wondering styles characterised via hobby to element, pattern popularity, and non-linear thinking. These cognitive strengths contribute to their trouble-fixing capabilities and functionality to approach stressful conditions from unconventional angles. They can choose out innovative answers and opportunity techniques that others might not with out problems don't forget. Autistic individuals' resilience lies in their capacity to count on outside the sector, adapt to new situations, and constantly look for powerful strategies to conquer limitations.

Supportive Networks and Social Connections:

Building supportive relationships and having a sturdy community of understanding individuals is critical for the resilience of autistic humans. These networks can consist of circle of relatives people, friends, educators, and specialists who offer emotional guide, guidance, and hotels. Autistic human beings who have a help tool that acknowledges their specific desires and fosters a splendid surroundings are higher ready to navigate annoying conditions. The presence of empathetic and accepting individuals lets in cultivate resilience via the use of imparting a experience of belonging and fostering an facts of their studies.

Adaptive Strategies and Coping Mechanisms:

Autistic people frequently boom adaptive strategies to control sensory sensitivities, verbal exchange problems, and social interactions. These strategies can include the use of seen enables, assistive technology, social scripts, or self-regulation techniques. By implementing those coping mechanisms, autistic human beings can navigate their environments extra efficaciously and decrease the impact of overwhelming sensory reports or tough social situations. The development and usage of these strategies are testaments to their resilience and capability to evolve to a international that won't continuously accommodate their unique dreams.

Emotional Regulation and Coping Skills:

Emotional regulation can be a huge undertaking for autistic humans due to sensory sensitivities, issues with social conversation, and heightened emotional research. However, many autistic human beings expand effective coping talents to govern their emotions and navigate overwhelming conditions. These coping mechanisms also can contain self-soothing strategies, assignment calming sports activities activities, or searching for help from trusted individuals. By developing emotional law strategies, autistic individuals can foster resilience and maintain their well-being, even in the face of emotional stressful conditions.

Overcoming Stigma and Advocating for Inclusion:

Autistic people regularly face societal stigma, misconceptions, and discrimination because of a lack of information of autism. However, many human beings with autism show off amazing resilience in hard societal norms and advocating for autism reputation and inclusion. Their perseverance lies in embracing their particular identification, tough stereotypes, and teaching others about autism. By actively contributing to public discourse and raising recognition, they try to create first-rate alternate and foster a greater inclusive society for themselves and destiny generations.

Personal Growth and Self-Acceptance:

Resilience and perseverance are cautiously tied to private increase and self-recognition.

Autistic those who domesticate self-reputation recognize their personal definitely well worth, embracing every their strengths and stressful conditions. They hobby on non-public increase, placing dreams, and working within the path of exciting their aspirations. This mind-set allows them to evolve to problems, observe from critiques, and maintain transferring ahead, even within the face of setbacks. Autistic folks that prioritize private increase and self-reputation growth a robust sense of resilience, allowing them to persevere and thrive regardless of demanding situations.

Chapter 12: Diagnostic Gear

The Modified Checklist for Autism in Toddlers (M-CHAT) – a questionnaire that can be administered to dad and mom of younger youngsters to evaluate social verbal exchange capabilities and conduct.

After a screening take a look at identifies a infant as being at chance for ASD, professionals use a more entire evaluation to confirm an ASD evaluation. Some common diagnostic tools embody:

The Autism Diagnostic InterviewRevised (ADI-R) – a semi-primarily based completely interview with primary caregivers that analyzes the kid's development, behavior styles, and language skills

The ADOS-2 – a standardized, semi-set up assessment that consists of a series of activities and obligations to evaluate social communique capabilities, stereotypical behaviors, and constrained pursuits.

The Childhood Autism Rating Scale (CARS) – a diagnostic score scale that evaluates social conversation talents, stereotypical behaviors, and limited hobbies.

Strengths and weaknesses of assessment tools

Each assessment tool has strengths and limitations, and specialists often use multiple device to make a analysis. For example, the M-CHAT is a beneficial screening tool but does no longer provide a analysis. ADOS-2 is an great tool for comparing social verbal exchange skills however may additionally additionally underneath-represent stereotypical behaviors if used on my own. The ADI-R can provide treasured statistics on a toddler's development and behavior statistics however can be time-ingesting to govern.

Personal critiques

One own family's experience with ASD evaluation and treatment highlights the significance of an correct and timely analysis. After noticing that their toddler became no longer meeting traditional developmental milestones, the own family sought out a prognosis from a pediatrician. The toddler have grow to be in the long run diagnosed with autism, and the family modified into stated a team of professionals who helped to growth a remedy plan that included in depth behavioral recuperation strategies. Despite initial stressful situations, the kid has made big development in phrases of verbal exchange, social interplay, and every day dwelling capabilities.

Importance of early evaluation and intervention

Research shows that early intervention can bring about higher results for children with ASD. Early diagnosis and treatment can assist decorate social communique, conduct, and educational results. It is crucial to are searching for assessment right away, as a do away with in analysis can result in overlooked opportunities for intervention.

Resources & Support for Individuals and Families Affected by the usage of manner of ASD

Families and those stricken by ASD can discover useful aid thru numerous neighborhood and countrywide groups. The Autism Society presents property and services, which encompass informational assets, help companies, and advocacy property. The Autism Speaks organization has a strong useful resource manual, which offers links to books, films, and apps designed for humans with ASD or their households. Additionally, close by network facilities, such as the YMCA and early intervention programs, frequently have sources and support groups to be had.

Know Your Rights: Laws and Autism

Know Your Rights: Laws and Autism

If you or your infant has autism, some of the most primary things you can have a observe and studies are your rights. Every American citizen is protected below the charter, and there are specific crook hints that have been surpassed to help protect people with autism and distinct disabilities.

By know-how the criminal guidelines that guard you or your autistic loved ones, you may stay in a international that offers better opportunities to each person, no matter not excellent incapacity, but moreover race, gender, and ethnicity. This is sincerely step one to growing a greater tolerant global in fashionable.

The first regulation with which you need to emerge as familiar is I.D.E.A., or the Individuals with Disabilities Education Act. The I.D.E.A. Covers kids a while three to 21 and gives autistic children with the unique educational programs they need.

The I.D.E.A. Offers parents the right to be involved with academic selections concerning their infant made via the university. Your little one first wants to be assessed to qualify below the I.D.E.A., and that is awesome completed by using a personal expert.

In the stop, your infant has the proper thru law to get keep of a loose public schooling that is appropriate for his or her talent degree. If your public faculty has no such utility, they may be required to find out one or create one for free of charge to you.

Also become acquainted with and informed about the American Disabilities Act. Under this act, discrimination due to incapacity is a criminal offense in the body of employees, in addition to with kingdom and community authorities, public motels, The United States Congress, public transportation, and telecommunications. For instance, in case you are autistic, however have the abilities to do a nice interest, you can't be refused the hobby due to your autism.

Other criminal suggestions offer rights for human beings with autism so that they're constitutionally same to others. One such law says that people with autism have the proper to vote, and accommodations need to be made in order that this is viable.

Another says that autistic individuals can't be refused housing primarily based mostly on disability. Others offer identical rights in all unique elements of lifestyles, and people have to specifically be studied if the one that you love with autism is in a fitness care institution.

By expertise the law and the way it applies to your self or others with autism, you could make certain that justice is upheld. If you have questions, nearby law officers need to be equipped and inclined to reply you or provide you with material to answer your very personal questions.

Remember that lack of awareness of the regulation is not a legitimate excuse for honestly all of us, so be an advocate for yourself or others with autism to prevent mistreatment.

Legal Rights and Protections for People on the Autism Spectrum: A Simple Guide

Introduction

Living with autism gives a totally specific set of worrying situations for human beings and their households. In addition to the social, emotional, and scientific annoying conditions that include autism, people at the autism spectrum face discrimination and exclusion from society.

However, there are legal pointers and hints in place to guard the rights of people with disabilities, consisting of autism. In this guide, we are able to communicate the legal rights and protections available to people on the autism spectrum and provide realistic recommendation on how to indicate for yourself or your beloved.

The Americans with Disabilities Act (ADA)

The Americans with Disabilities Act (ADA) is a federal law that prohibits discrimination in competition to individuals with disabilities.

Autism is taken into consideration a incapacity under the ADA, and those on the autism spectrum are entitled to the identical rights and protections as unique human beings with disabilities. The ADA protects people with autism from discrimination in employment, housing, public accommodations, and different regions of life.

Employment: Employers can not discriminate in opposition to people with autism within the hiring, firing, or advertising manner. Employers ought to moreover offer reasonable accommodation, such as modified paintings schedules or hobby schooling, for personnel with autism to perform their mission duties.

Housing: Landlords can't discriminate closer to human beings with autism while renting or selling housing. They need to additionally permit low-price accommodations, which consist of enterprise animals, for individuals with autism.

Public resorts: Individuals with autism have the right to get proper of access to public places, which encompass restaurants, shops, and authorities homes, without facing discrimination or barriers to get right of access to.

Public motels have to additionally offer low-fee inns, consisting of wheelchair ramps or sensory-exceptional environments, for humans with autism to get entry to their offerings.

The Individuals with Disabilities Education Act (IDEA)The Individuals with Disabilities Education Act (IDEA) is a federal regulation that ensures a loose and suitable public training (FAPE) for kids with disabilities from ages three to 21 years antique.

Children with autism are entitled to an individualized training plan (IEP) that outlines their training dreams and lodges. The IDEA additionally calls for colleges to offer associated offerings, together with speech and occupational remedy, to children with autism.

Advocating for Yourself or Your Loved One

Knowing your rights and advocating for your self or your beloved is vital in making sure identical possibilities and protection. Here are some sensible pointers for advocating for your self or the one that you love:

-Know your rights underneath the ADA and IDEA and be knowledgeable about the prison guidelines and guidelines that shield human beings with autism.

-Develop a guide network of specialists, advocates, and own family those who can help in advocating for you or the one you love.

-Communicate efficaciously with schools, employers, and public motels to say your rights and request lodges while important.

Seek criminal assist or document a criticism with the nice organization, alongside side the

Equal Employment Opportunity Commission or the Department of Education, in case your rights have been violated.

Resources for Support and Information

There are many assets available for humans and households dwelling with autism. Here are a few companies and web websites that offer guide and data:

-Autistic Self Advocacy Network (ASAN): This corporation advocates

for the inclusion and rights of people with autism.

-National Autism Association (NAA): This business enterprise offers aid and belongings for households suffering from autism.

-Autism Society: This employer increases reputation and offers help for human beings and households tormented by autism.

-Disability Rights Education and Defense Fund (DREDF): This organisation business enterprise offers prison assist and assets for humans with disabilities.

Living with autism gives its very own specific set of demanding situations, however there are felony suggestions and policies in vicinity to defend the rights of human beings with disabilities, which includes autism. The ADA and IDEA offer important protections for human beings with autism, and advocating for your self or the one you love is vital in making sure their identical opportunities and protections. There are also many assets to be had for resource and information. By understanding your rights and

Advocating for your self or your loved one, people with autism can lead fascinating lives free from discrimination and limitations to get right of entry to.

Chapter 13: Busting The Autism Stereotypes

Busting the Autism Stereotypes

As with every person with a bodily or intellectual disease, autistic humans address a sizeable variety of reactions from others, from entire assist to uncaring lack of expertise.

Unfortunately, even those who help autistic family individuals, co-employees, and buddies might not apprehend autism very well. This effects in stereotypes, that would result in hatred, embarrassment, or different unhappy conditions. By becoming informed about autism, you can help others in your network deal with this illness.

It is most vital to word that not all autistic human beings are the equal. Other ailments and issues have their very own gadgets of regulations, but autism is this type of complicated clinical situation, that everyone reacts in another manner to it.

Autistic human beings are generally rated on a functional scale, with immoderate-functioning humans being able to preserve jobs and coffee-functioning humans wanting 24-hour-a-day care.

Symptoms embody behavioral challenges, uncontrollable movements, speech and conversation problems, and emotional inadequacies. Some show all symptoms and signs, whilst one-of-a-kind show few, and though others may moreover furthermore have maximum below manage to the detail in which you can not tell they have got autism in any respect.

Because all and sundry is one among a type, no individual detail can be stated approximately autism and be actual ordinary. However, maximum autistic human beings have trouble talking feelings. This does no longer advocate that an autistic man or woman does not experience.

He or she truly can't specific this feel. It also does now not suggest robust courting bonds are not viable. On the alternative, many autistic people are fortuitously married and in love. Forming relationships is more tough for maximum however can be carried out over the years.

Many humans agree with that being autistic coincides with being a genius in some issue. While it's miles proper that some autistic humans have top notch math, song, and art competencies, this variety is nowhere close to the majority-in fact, especially few autistic humans function outside of the everyday range in any capacity.

This stereotype is perpetuated inside the movies and on tv, due to the fact the tale of a professional person stopping terrible elements (collectively with autism) makes an exceptional plot.

However, this isn't the norm, so nothing greater than the splendid they might in my view do should be anticipated from an autistic man or woman. However, it is critical to look at that autism isn't always a form of intellectual retardation. Some autistic humans are mentally retarded as well, however maximum aren't and want to not be handled as such.

In the give up, the maximum vital lesson to cast off from your research on autism is considered one of tolerance.

You will probably want to be affected person while dealing with autistic people, however through understanding a chunk greater approximately the sickness, probably this could be much less tough. Learn what you may and unfold the understanding to those you understand to assist create a extra tolerant putting for autistic people on your network.

Autism has extended been shrouded in stereotypes and misconceptions. The portrayal of autism in the media and well-known manner of existence has often been one-dimensional, depicting individuals with autism as both savants or non-communicative humans with out a social abilties. These stereotypes have brought about a loss of facts and reputation of human beings with autism, and regularly make contributions to discrimination and exclusion.

One not unusual misconception is that autism is due to terrible parenting or a lack of love and affection. This has been debunked through manner of numerous research that have validated that autism is a neurodevelopmental sickness that is essentially genetic. While environmental elements can make a contribution to the improvement of autism, they'll be now not the primary motive.

Another dangerous stereotype is that people with autism lack empathy and social abilties. This in reality is not real. While people with autism also can moreover warfare with social interactions and communication, they'll be despite the fact that able to empathy and forming significant connections with others. In fact, many humans with autism have a heightened revel in of empathy and are greater attuned to the feelings of others.

Additionally, the trope of the "autistic genius" is not representative of anyone with autism. While a few human beings with autism can also have exceptional abilities in certain areas, such as math or track, this is not the case for all and sundry. Many people with autism have not unusual or below not unusual intelligence, and conflict with duties that others may also additionally discover clean.

Personal recollections and reviews from people with autism and their families are important in imparting a human perspective on autism. These memories can help venture stereotypes and misconceptions and showcase the diversity of research and abilties within the autism community.

One person who has shared their experience with autism is Dr. Temple Grandin, a well-known autism propose and professor of animal technology. Grandin, who became identified with autism as a little one, has spoken publicly approximately how her autism has original her life and career. She has additionally spoken approximately the importance of know-how and accepting the variations that come with autism.

Another important voice inside the autism network is John Elder Robison, author of "Look Me within the Eye: My Life with Asperger's". Robison has spoken about the demanding situations he faced growing up with undiagnosed Asperger's syndrome, and the stigma he faced because of his differences.

It's time to project these stereotypes and misconceptions approximately autism. We want to apprehend that humans with autism are individuals with particular evaluations and views and should be dealt with with recognize and facts. This method growing extra inclusive groups, schools, and offices that accommodate the desires of human beings with autism and recognizing their fee and contributions.

We can start through tough our non-public biases and assumptions about autism and coaching ourselves at the actual nature of the ailment. We also can help autism advocacy agencies and autism research tasks, and paintings to promote recognition and inclusion of all individuals on the autism spectrum.

By doing so, we're able to create a more compassionate and information worldwide for people with autism and their households. Let's paintings toward building a global in which variations are celebrated, and all people are valued for who they may be.

My Child is Autistic-and I do now not Know what to Do...

My Child is Autistic-and I do not Know what to Do...

Discovering your infant has autism can be a distressing ordeal, and lamentably, time is of the essence. As a decide, you do now not have the time to don't forget why or how this took place, great what to do next.

The maximum critical component to take into account is which you aren't by myself in your struggle. By gaining knowledge of the disorder and locating others going through similar situations, you can assist your infant even as notwithstanding the truth that managing your very personal emotional reaction.

Join a help organization for parents with autism. You can discover those thru contacting the countrywide Autism Society of America. From there you can discover close by branches, loads of which provide manual corporations for parents and families with an autistic infant.

Being in contact with other mother and father in a comparable state of affairs can not only help you sense plenty much less by myself, however it is able to offer you with a myriad of property. A determine assist business enterprise can also even assist thing you within the course of the incredible clinical medical doctors, intervention programs, and workshops for both your toddler and your own family.

Find a guide group for some other children you've got were given as well. Many dad and mom forget about that they're no longer the great ones who must discover ways to live and speak with an autistic toddler. By locating a aid institution on your unique kids, you can help them from appearing out or performing in the direction of the autistic toddler with the resource of using education them about the contamination. As a parent, you want to create a supportive environment for the complete own family to properly manipulate your little one's infection.

Consider marriage counseling in case you are married. An autistic infant can positioned critical strain on a wedding, main to escalating arguments, overlook approximately of each different, or maybe probably blaming each other for the scenario. Marriage counseling from the very beginning can help a pair thru this discovery and hard transition and help bring together a higher supportive environment to your children.

Your marriage need to now not quit due to having an autistic toddler, but the unhappy truth is that plenty of them do. Prevent this with the resource of the utilization of each exclusive for assist and with the beneficial aid of information that you could want assist to cope with every other now and inside the future.

Most importantly, begin at the route to turning into an expert. Many times, pediatricians or psychiatrists aren't professionals on autism, which could result in incorrect diagnoses or wrong treatment options.

As your little one's pleasant recommend, you ought to recognize everything you could about autism. Parents of Autistic Children may be a exceptional resource; this company gives education and workshops. The ASA has a manual and offers a number of facts, from diagnosing to treating.

As normally, recall that a resource group of parents with autistic youngsters can constantly offer you with books and studies that specializes in the fact of the situation. Educate your self and people around you to provide the most useful topics on your infant-love and guidance.

Being a determine of an autistic infant comes with a variety of worrying situations and testimonies that others can also in no manner completely apprehend. From the immediate my little one turned into diagnosed, my worldwide modified, and I had to alter to a present day truth of parenting.

Obtaining a prognosis come to be a protracted and difficult technique that required infinite appointments, testing, and opinions. It have become tough to just accept that my infant had a scenario that we knew little or no approximately, however we knew that early intervention have become essential to their fulfillment.

Finding assets and help for our infant became every other undertaking we confronted. We needed to navigate through a good sized variety of services and packages, frequently with masses of prepared lists and limited belongings. But, over time, we built a community of specialists, therapists, and distinct mother and father who have been going thru comparable critiques, and that manual made all of the difference.

Identifying the simplest remedy alternatives for my infant became additionally hard. We tried diverse treatments and strategies, and in the end, we discovered what labored first-class for our little one. We decided that each toddler with autism is specific and calls for an individualized method to treatment.

Through our adventure with autism, we've got located out so much, and we want to share our enjoy with others.

Here are some practical recommendations and strategies that have worked for us:

1. Learn as an lousy lot as feasible approximately autism. Understanding the signs and symptoms and symptoms and signs, signs and symptoms and signs, and treatment options will help you advise in your toddler and make knowledgeable alternatives.

2. Build a assist community. Connect with different parents, experts, and agencies that offer help and assets for households with autistic kids.

3. Consider distinctive treatments and interventions. What works for one infant won't artwork for some other, so it is critical to have an open mind and strive specific strategies.

four. Create regular sporting events on your little one. Autistic kids thrive on shape and predictability, and putting in place regular exercise routines can offer them with a revel in of comfort and protection.

five. Practice splendor and inclusion. It's essential to recognize that autism isn't a sickness or a few element to treatment; it's a totally specific way of being that calls for reputation and data.

It's essential to cope with a number of the commonplace misconceptions and stereotypes surrounding autism. Autistic people aren't all of the equal; they have unique personalities, capabilities, and traumatic conditions. It's important to recognize and embody their variations and strengths and now not pick out them based totally on stereotypes and assumptions.

Our wish for our toddler's destiny is that society turns into greater accepting and which embody autistic people. We preference that they may have opportunities to live exciting lives, acquire their complete ability, and participate in society without going through discrimination or stigma.

In end, being a parent of an autistic little one is tough, however it has additionally been a journey of exceptional boom and reading. We preference that sharing our reviews and insights can assist one of a kind parents navigate this journey and assist society become extra accepting and on the aspect of the autistic network.

A Gift of Sight: Visual Perception Treatment for Autistic Children

A Gift of Sight: Visual Perception Treatment for Autistic Children

Autism impacts every infant in a different way, so it's far tough to discover the first-rate remedies your toddler desires to deal with his or her signs and signs and symptoms.

One element that influences a few autistic kids (regardless of the fact that, not all) is problems with seen belief. By the use of a few standardized strategies to assist beautify seen notion, you could offer your child the capacity to see the arena greater virtually, making reading and comprehension much less complex and probably curbing a few conduct issues as nicely.

Autistic kids in particular have issues with sensory overload and distortion. These are some of the same problems many humans now not tormented by the disorder enlarge, and so many treatment options have turn out to be to be had.

Individuals with autism often discover, however, that the sensory overload of the arena due to mild, hues, assessment, shapes, and patterns, is too much to deal with, causing them to behave out or near down in stylish.

This is now and again a genetic state of affairs that is without a doubt more potent via autism, so if the kid's dad and mom have hassle with analyzing or were in any other case handled for visible perceptive troubles, there's a top notch risk that the kid dreams assist as nicely.

The Irene Method is one powerful manner to cope with seen belief troubles. This method makes use of color to create a more harmonized international.

You might also moreover have heard of these strategies if every person has ever recommended using a color clean out over the internet net web page at the same time as reading as a way to observe better and extra speedy. This approach is tested to art work, and in case your autistic little one is on the adulthood degree of analyzing, you can want to try the ones shade filters to see if there may be a difference in pace and comprehension.

However, it's far much more likely that your autistic little one will gain from colour filters during the whole day, not absolutely on the same time as reading. Special glasses have been made the usage of colored lenses to conquer this trouble.

Not each child responds the equal manner to each color, so it is a manner of trial and mistakes to find out which color is the fine blocking the damaging slight. You also can pick out to use colored slight bulbs in your private home to help autistic individuals with their visible perception issues.

This technique in particular helps youngsters in four regions: depth perception, social interplay, mastering, and physical nicely-being. The colorations help the child decide how a long manner he or she is from an object, and the area turns into greater 3-dimensional, assisting depth belief.

Social interplay additionally improves due to the reality the child feels as despite the reality that he or she is in a calmer global and might greater truely see and interpret facial expressions. The shades make it viable to observe, especially when reading, and common, the child will revel in higher, because it allows reduce complications and dizziness.